KETO INSTANT POT COOKBOOK

500+ Wholesome Recipes You'll Want to Make Everyday.

The Complete Guide to Keto Diet Instant Pot Cooking for Beginners to Improve Your Health and to Lose Weight!

Cover design by Olivia Rhodes
Interior design by Nigel Barnett

The Publisher publishes its books in a variety of electronic, audio and print formats. Some content that appears in print may not be available in electronic or audio books, and vice versa.

ISBN 9798614231699

Table of contents

Introduction

My story has started a long time before I decided to be slim. Ever since childhood, I was overweight. During the teen time, my situation wasn't so deplorable. I am grateful to my family because they always accepted me as I am. But it wasn't enough for me because all around hated me. At the age of 15, I understood that I am unshapely girl. I was in graduation class, my weight has already exceeded 270 lbs. I felt like I am a giant cow who couldn't fit into any sexy dress for a prom party. My parents have never been worried about weight, they just repeated all the time "you are an angel, you are beautiful". I knew that it wasn't true, in the mirror I saw plum girl. After graduating from school, I became very depressed. All my troubles I jammed with tones of chocolate and Coke.

One sunny day I firmly decided for myself - enough for me! I don't want to live like that anymore. I will be changed. I had made the "wish map", where I was slim and smiling, and started to do sports and eat fewer sweets and sparkling drinks. I couldn't say that it wasn't successful but I didn't get the desired result. I wanted everything at once, so I even practiced fasting. I could drink water and vegetable smoothies for 2-3 days. But it all ended with me breaking down and gaining even more weight. At that time, I already started having health problems. I could not walk for a long time, I was haunted by headaches, pain in my stomach, as well as bad breath.

I decided to go to the doctor and do a comprehensive analysis of the whole body. When my doctor looked at my tests, he advised going to a nutritionist. This time I discovered a ketogenic diet. The doctor didn't prescribe something special. It was a certain diet and simple physical exercises every day. But I have to eat a lot of proteins, and almost no vegetables (I hated them at that time). I couldn't believe that everything is so easy! But I didn't lose faith and clearly followed the doctor's instructions. After a week of keto life, I did not see significant results, but after 2 weeks the arrows of the scales showed -8 lbs. During the year of keto lifestyle, my weight dropped by 83 lbs and my health became better. I cried with happiness! Finally, I did it! This is just a miracle! Now I am a wife, mom, and just happy woman!

I wrote this book to help people like me. To those who still think that they are hopeless! I am sure that this diet will change your way of thinking and make a big difference in your life. I am the greatest example that nothing is impossible. You should know that losing weight is not only restrictions and starving. The real-life on keto diet exists and this book proves it! Our mind and our body are omnipotent! They know well what we need! Each of us should be dropkicked to take the path of a happy life! I strongly believe that this book will be a guide and silver lining in a better version of you!

What to Eat and Avoid on the Keto Diet

Meat and poultry
Actually, it is the primary type of food for the Keto diet. It contains 0% of carbs and is rich in potassium, selenium, zinc, and B vitamins. Grass-fed meat and poultry are the most beneficial. It caused by high omega 3 fats and antioxidants content. Bear in mind that Keto diet is a high-fat diet and high consumption of proteins can cause to harder getting of ketosis.

What to eat	Enjoy occasionally	What to avoid
- chicken - duck - goose - ground beef - lamb - ostrich - partridge - pheasant - pork - quail - turkey - venison	- bacon - ham - low-fat meat, such as skinless chicken breast - sausage	- breaded meats - processed meats

Dairy
High-fat dairy products are awesome for the keto diet. They are calcium-rich full-fat dairy product is nutritious and can make you full longer. Milk lovers should restrict or even cross out this product from the daily meal plan. It is allowed only 1 tablespoon of milk in your drink per day but doesn't abuse it daily.

What to eat	What to avoid
- butter - cheese (soft and hard) - full-fat yogurt - heavy cream - sour cream	- fat-free yogurt - low-fat cheese - milk - skim milk - skim mozzarella - sweetened yogurt

Fish and Seafood
Fatty fish as salmon is beneficial for the keto diet. Small fish like sardines, herring, etc. are less in toxins. The best option for a keto diet is wild-caught seafood; it has a higher number of omega 3 fats. Scientifically proved that frequent eating of fish improves mental health.

What to eat	Enjoy occasionally	What to avoid
- catfish - clams - cod - crab - halibut - herring - lobster - mackerel - Mahi Mahi - mussels - oysters	- prawns - salmon - sardines - scallops - shrimp - snapper - swordfish - tilapia - trout - tuna	- breaded fish

Nuts and Seeds

These products are heart-healthy and fiber-rich. Nevertheless, eat nuts and seeds as a snack is a bad idea. As usual, the amount of eaten food can be much more than allowed. Nuts like cashews are very insidious and contain a lot of carbohydrates. Replace them with macadamia or pecan.

What to eat		What to avoid
- almonds	- peanuts	- cashews
- chia seeds	- pecans	- pistachio
- flaxseeds	- pumpkin seeds	- chocolate-covered nuts
- hazelnuts	- walnuts	- nut butter (sweetened)
- nut butter (unsweetened)	- macadamia nuts	

Oils and fats

It is the main component of the keto-friendly sauces and dressings.

Olive oil and coconut oil are highly recommending for everyone who decided to follow the keto diet. They are almost perfect it their fatty acid composition. Avoid artificial trans fats which are poison for our body. This type of fats, as usual, used in French fries, margarine, and crackers.

What to eat		What to avoid	
- avocado oil	- pumpkin seed oil	- grapeseed oil	- peanut oil
- coconut oil	- sesame oil	- canola oil	- soybean oil
- hazelnut oil	- walnut oil	- cottonseed oil	- safflower oil
- olive oil		- hydrogenated oils	- processed vegetable oils
		- margarine	

Vegetables

Keto diet cannot work without vegetables, but their usage should be in moderation. Starchy vegetables such as potatoes, sweet potatoes, etc. are deadly for our body and will not bring anything more than overweight. At the same time, vegetables that are low in carbs, are rich in antioxidants and can protect the body from free radicals that damage our cells.

What to eat		What to avoid	
- asparagus	- mushrooms	- carrots	- pumpkin
- avocado	- olives	- corn	- turnips
- broccoli	- onions	- beets	- yams
- cabbage	- tomatoes	- butternut squash	- yuca
- cauliflower	- peppers	- parsnips	- other starchy vegetables
- celery	- spinach	- potatoes (both sweet and regular)	
- cucumber	- zucchini		
- eggplant	- other nonstarchy vegetables		
- leafy greens			
- lettuce			

Fruits

This type of food is high in carbs that's why they should be limited while keto diet. Besides this, almost all fruits are high in glucose and can enhance blood sugar.

Enjoy occasionally	What to avoid	
- lemons	- apples	- peaches
- pomegranates	- bananas	- pears
- limes	- grapefruits	- pineapple
	- limes	- plums
	- mango	- dried fruits
	- oranges	

Berries

If you are looking for how to substitute fruits, this is your godsend. Berries contain up to 12 grams of net carbs per 3.5 ounces serving. They are high in fiber and can maintain the health of your body and fight with diseases. Note consumption of a huge amount of berries can be harmful.

What to eat		What to avoid	
- blackberries	- raspberries	- cherries	- melon
- blueberries	- strawberries	- grapes	- watermelon

Eggs

This is the most wholesome food in the world. Use them everywhere you want! Containing less than one gram of carbohydrates, eggs are a wonderful food for the keto lifestyle. Eating eggs reducing the risk of heart disease and save your eyes health.

Note: free-range eggs are healthier options for the keto diet.

What to eat	
- chicken eggs	- ostrich eggs
- duck eggs	- quail eggs
- goose eggs	

Condiments

Condiments can make any type of meal awesome. Even a piece of meat will turn into the masterpiece with them. There are only a few products which are better to avoid; nevertheless, nowadays, you can find keto-friendly substitutors in a supermarket.

One more hot tip: putting hot pepper in your meal will reduce the amount of salt you need and make the taste of the dish more saturated.

What to eat	What to avoid
- herbs and spices	- BBQ sauce
- lemon juice	- hot sauces
- mayonnaise with no added sugar	- ketchup
- salad dressings with no added sugar	- maple syrup
- salt and pepper	- salad dressings with added sugar
- vinegar	- sweet dipping sauces
	- tomato sauce

Grain products

Actually, it is needless to say that all grains are forbidden and can't be eaten if you want to achieve ketosis. Grains contain complex carbohydrates that have a feature to be absorbed slower than simple carbohydrates. For better understanding, if the food has keto-friendly carbs, look at the number of starch and sugar. Their number should be minimum.

What to avoid			
- baked goods	- crackers	- oats	- rice
- bread	- flour	- pasta	- wheat
- cereal	- granola	- pizza	
- corn	- muesli	- popcorn	

Beans and legumes

There are no ingredients in this food group that would be healthy for a keto diet. Beans and legumes contain fewer carbs in comparison with root vegetables such as potatoes; nevertheless, this type of carbohydrates fastly adds up.

What to avoid			
- black beans	- kidney beans	- navy beans	- pinto beans
- chickpeas	- lentils	- peas	- soybeans

Beverages

A variety of keto drinks may shock you. Probably you know that the best beverage for a keto diet is water. Nevertheless, in order to brighten up a little gray everyday life of keto lovers, the consumption of alcoholic beverages is allowed in moderation. For instance, pure forms of alcohol, such as gin, vodka, or tequila can be drunk once per week. They contain zero amounts of carbs. Avoid all sweetened beverages; they are a priori high carbohydrate.

What to drink	Enjoy occasionally	What to avoid
- almond milk	- dry wine	- alcoholic drinks
- bone broth	- hard liquor	(sweetened)
- coffee (unsweetened)	- vodka	- beer
- flax milk	- other low carb alcoholic	- cider
- tea (unsweetened)	drinks	- coffee (sweetened)
- water (still and sparkling)		- fruit juice
		- soda
		- sports drinks
		- smoothies
		- tea (sweetened)
		- wines (sweet)

Sweets

Cakes and cookies cannot help in losing weight in any diet. As for keto, here everything is strict with this. You should try to avoid sugar and sweeteners in any form. Moreover, sweets negatively affect blood sugar and insulin levels.

Enjoy occasionally	What to avoid	
- erythritol	- artificial sweeteners	- ice cream
- stevia	- buns	- pastries
- sucralose	- candy	- pies
	- cakes	- pudding
	- chocolate	- sugar
	- cookies	- tarts
	- custard	

Others

Fast food and processed food contain a huge amount of stabilizers and harmful carbohydrates. The main rule of the Keto diet is avoiding sugar. 99,9% of such food contains harmful sugars. The existence of which in the body negates the achievement of ketosis.

What to avoid
- fast food
- processed foods

TOP 10 Instant Pot Tips

1. Flavored liquids enhance your meal.

Broths, juices, dairies, and stocks can enhance the taste of your meal. This kind of liquids has the property not only to convey its taste but also the taste of spices that were used while cooking. Don't be afraid of experiments! The mixture of chicken beef broth and sautéed garlic instead of ordinary water will turn the lean rice on a flavored meal.

2. Cook by small pieces instead of the whole product.

You can reduce the cooking time almost two times by chopping the ingredients into small pieces. Doing this, the pressure and steam will reach the ingredients evenly and will cook them faster.

3. Make the sauces and gravies after cooking.

Thickening liquids is a good way to get delicious gravies; they can improve the taste of your dish. The best liquid thickeners are starch and flour. Adding them in the last minutes of cooking will make the texture of the meal more saturated and uniform. Also, this method helps not to overcook the ingredients, do not deprive them of vitamins and as a result, make the food healthier.

4. A steaming rack is a good option for any meal.

Almost all Instant pot models come with steamer rack that is essential not only for cooking vegetables. This tool can be appropriate at any time when you want to cook the ingredients with less amount of liquids. Such food as pies, fish, or meat will have a completely different taste if you use steamer rack while cooking.

5. Use improvised things.

Nowadays, the market suggests a huge variety of accessories for instant pot. Some of them have important meaning but some can be substitute by simple things. For instance, foil can be a wonderful replacement for instant pot trays and molds. It can take any form and has non-stick features. Use it for cooking muffins, pies, and even meatloaves.

6. Cooking with pressure can take more time.

As a rule, it takes approximately 10-15 minutes to reach the needed pressure in the inner pot. Very rarely the recipes include this time in the total cooking time; that's to accurately determine the cooking time and notify your family when it is time to eat, add extra minutes to the cooking time specified in the recipe.

7. Cook two or more meals per one time.

The instant pot comes with only one inner pot, which is not always convenient when cooking several dishes. Therefore, nimble housewives found an excellent life hack on how to save time not only on cooking but also on washing dishes. To do this, simply purchase a few more inner pots and cook meals more quickly.

8. Get rid of odors.

Using the sealing rings will help you to avoid the odors. As usual, the smell of spices after cooking meat, fish, or vegetable meals are very strong. That's why it is highly recommended to buy extra sealing rings for all the most popular types of meal you cook; so each dish can retain its unique taste and flavor.

9. Easy cleaning.

Use a dishwasher to wash all removable parts of the instant pot. Detergent and a strong flow of water in the dishwasher will make your instant pot clean and at the same time save your time. For non-removable instant pot parts, use vinegar and lemon juice. They can make your kitchen appliance sparkle like new.

10. Clean nooks, so instant pot is always like new.

Sometimes the nooks of instant pot become clogged with sauces, steam after using pressure cooking mode or food leftovers that were accidentally spilled. Clean the nooks with the help of the brush and paper after each usage of the instant pot to preserve its original appearance for many years.

Top 10 Keto Diet Tips

1. **Combine together Keto and Intermittent fasting.**

Intermittent fasting (IF) is the right way to get ketosis. It gives your body additional benefits.

Scientists showed that connection keto diet and intermittent fasting can up the results which can give only strict following of the keto diet.

IF means not eating and drinking during a determined amount of time. It is recommended to separate your day into a building phase (BP) and cleansing phase(CP); where the building phase is the time between the first and last time of eating (first-last); and cleansing is the opposite time (last-first). Start from 14-hours CP and 11-hours BP. Continue like this till your body adapts to the new daily plan. It can take 2-3 days. The first days will be the hardest but then you will feel relief and you can safely proceed to the next stage where BP turns into 5 hours and CP - into 19 hours.

According to research, women get the highest benefits of IF. It is possible to get rid of adrenal fatigue, hypothyroid, and hormonal imbalance.

2. **Staying hydrated is essential.**

Our body is 60% water. Water ensures the normal digestion of food and the absorption of nutrients from the intestines. If there is not enough water in the body, there will be discomfort in the abdomen and constipation. Drinking water is important even if you are not on keto.

The kidneys filter 5,000 ounces of blood per day so that the result is 50 ounces of urine. For the normal elimination of toxins and waste substances, you need to drink at least 50 ounces of water per day, but preferably more.

Many people face the problem of unwillingness to drink water. The best way to prevent dehydration and all its unpleasant consequences is to put a bottle or cup of water on the table and take a sip every time you look at the water. If you realize that you are thirsty, then eliminate thirst in time.

Regular drinking of the right amount of water for 1 week will become a habit and you will not be able to live differently.

3. **Salt isn't harmful.**

Salt plays an important role in complex metabolic processes. It is part of the blood, lymph, saliva, tears, gastric juice, bile - that is, all the fluids of our body. Any fluctuations in the salt content in the blood plasma lead to serious metabolic disorders

When fewer carbohydrates enter the body, insulin levels drop. Less insulin circulating in the body leads to secrete excess water in the kidneys instead of holding it. It means that salt and other important minerals and electrolytes are washed out of the body.

Replenish salt is possible by eating bone broths, cucumbers, celeriac, salty keto nuts, and seeds.

The best salts for keto diet are 2 types of salt. Pink salt has a more saturated, saltier taste, and contains calcium, magnesium, and potassium. Sea salt is simply evaporated seawater. The crystals of sea salt are slightly larger than iodized salt, and it has a stronger aroma. It contains potassium, magnesium, sulfur, phosphorus, and zinc.

4. **Sport is important.**

It is proved that physical activity improves the health of the whole body in general and accelerates metabolism. When we do sport, the first thing is we get rid of carbohydrates, and only then we burn fats.

On a keto diet, even minimal physical activity contributes to the rapid decomposition of fats. You simply don't have glucose (carbohydrates) and any load breaks down fats. The most effective workouts on an empty stomach. Sports during keto are very comfortable. You do not feel hungry and can play sports without breakdowns and overeating. Your stamina is significantly increased. If the protein is correctly calculated, you don't lose muscle mass with a calorie deficit.

The combination of three types of workouts gives the best result for health, weight dynamics, and even mood! These are workouts, aerobic, and stretching. Start with small loads every day and increase it as you can. Do not forget to take measurements of your body to monitor the result!

5. Reduce stress.

Sometimes, observing all the postulates of the keto lifestyle, ketosis does not occur or occurs very slowly. In 99 cases, it happens due to the level of stress in your life. Thus, the hormone cortisol rises, the sympathetic nervous system is stimulated.

Cortisol is produced in response to any stress, even the most minor. How does it happen?

Cortisol "eats" our muscles to turn them into glucose, it catabolizes bones, which is fraught with osteoporosis, causes increased appetite, and suppresses immunity. It also causes increased production of glucose and insulin, and exactly this stops ketosis.

During keto-adaptation (the first 3 weeks), increased cortisol is produced, because the usual energy, glucose, ceases to flow into the body, and it turns on the "self-preservation mode".

It is very important at first to minimize stress from the outside, then everything will normalize.

You should be able to switch from stimulation of the sympathetic nervous system to parasympathetic. Stimulation of the parasympathetic nervous system contributes to the restoration and accumulation of energy resources. This can be achieved by a simple 15 minutes' meditation. The time when you cannot be interrupted.

6. Sleep above all!

Sleep and stress are two interconnected components. Lack of sleep leads to increased stress. Consequently, stress hormone levels and blood sugar levels rise and we gain weight very fast.

Doctors recommend an 8-9 hour sleep every day. The best time to fall asleep is before 11 pm. An hour before bedtime, try not to use any gadgets. It is better to spend this time in silence, meditation, listening to calm music or reading a paper book. Thus, we calm the nervous system and set it to sleep. If your stress level per day was high, try to spend more time sleeping. it is the sleep that contributes to our weight loss and getting rid of all diseases. There are some tips to improve your sleep comfort:
- Keep cool in the room. The optimum temperature should not exceed 65-70F.
- Use a black mask for sleeping and earplugs.
- Provide good room ventilation.

7. Don't forget about vegetables.

It is obvious that the main resource of vitamins and minerals is vegetables. You can't cross out them totally from daily meals. Consuming them during the keto diet is very important, but should be in moderation. Starchy vegetables such as sweet potatoes and potatoes are not allowed. Nevertheless, at the same time, you can safely substitute them with broccoli, kale, spinach, white cabbage, Brussels sprouts to your diet. Such vegetables are not only low-carb, but also low-calorie and have a huge number of vitamins, antioxidants, and minerals. They will help you stay full for a long time and protect from eating an extra serving of nuts.

One of the tips of keto coaches is to pamper yourself with low-carb berries once a week. At the same time, it is very important to increase physical activity during this day. Cycling will be just right. All this will fill your body with useful antioxidants and will not add extra pounds.

8. MCT oil is a treasure for a keto diet.

MCT oil is medium-chain triglyceride oil. It practically doesn't require splitting in the small intestine and is absorbed already in the duodenum, going directly to the liver. MCT oil is used by the body as an energy source, which leads to an increase in fat loss. On the other hand, MCT oil isn't deposited in body fat like fatty tissue in comparison with other fatty acids, and it has been shown that it improves thermogenesis, that is, the process during which the body creates heat using excess energy.

MCT oils are good for cooking, especially for baking, frying or grilling. This is due to their high point of "smoke", which means that they are very difficult to oxidize from heat and can withstand high temperatures without losing their original chemical structure at room temperature (losing their useful properties). You can also add MTC oil in keto shakes, coffee, tea, and other keto drinks.

9. Do a kitchen audit

The key to getting ketosis is proper low-carb nutrition. Nevertheless, our brain, knowing that somewhere in the fridge or freezer are a bar of chocolate or a package of vanilla ice cream. So it unconsciously creates situations in which we are obliged to eat them. That's why there are no doubts that one of the best tips is to clean your kitchen and all the shelves from the "seducers". Firstly, write a list of food that is not allowed during the diet, and then one by one throw away everything that is on your list. It may seem too radical right away. But just know that all this will help you completely switch to keto life faster and less stressfully for your body. Also, you can make a list of all you have in the fridge and stick this sheet of paper on the fridge. Doing this you will not eat extra snacks during the day.

10. Keep food near you.

Our life is full of events and sometimes we just don't have time to cook. We have a choice to buy high carbohydrate food in the shop or cook the right food by ourselves. All of this needs extra time. That's why you should always have a "healthy snack" with you. No matter what it is. It can be fat bombs, seeds, or nuts. If you have more time, make the keto salads, or find the keto fruits such as avocado and cook the spreads and dips. But bear in mind, you shouldn't cook much in advance. Their expired date is very short. Follow the rule to purchasing all ingredients for snacks in advance, so that they are always in your fridge. This way you can less likely break your diet and get rid of unnecessary overeating. If you don't know what to cook, use the recipe generator which can help you with the meal for your certain list of food.

Breakfast

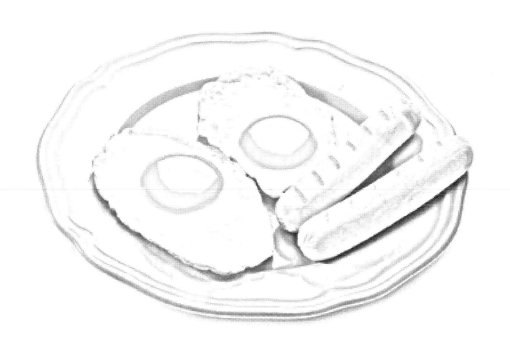

Breakfast Casserole

Prep time: 10 minutes | **Cook time:** 20 minutes | **Yield:** 6 servings

Ingredients

- 1 cup ground chicken
- 1 cup Cheddar cheese, shredded
- ½ cup coconut cream
- 1 teaspoon salt
- 1 teaspoon chili flakes
- 1 teaspoon olive oil

Method

1. Preheat the instant pot on Manual mode for 3 minutes.
2. Then add olive oil, ground chicken, salt, and chili flakes.
3. Cook the ground chicken on Saute mode for 10 minutes.
4. Then stir it well and add coconut cream and Cheddar cheese.
5. Close the lid and cook the casserole on Manual mode (high pressure) for 10 minutes. Then make a quick pressure release and let the meal cool for 10 minutes.

Nutritional info per serve: calories 173, fat 13.5, fiber 0.4, carbs 1.4, protein 11.9

Eggs Benedict

Prep time: 10 minutes | **Cook time:** 1 minute | **Yield:** 3 servings

Ingredients

- 3 eggs
- 3 turkey bacon slices, fried
- 1 teaspoon butter
- ½ teaspoon ground black pepper
- 1 cup of water
- ¼ teaspoon salt

Method

1. Grease the eggs molds with butter and crack eggs inside.
2. Sprinkle them with ground black pepper and salt.
3. Pour water in the instant pot and insert the rack.
4. Then place the eggs in the molds in the rack and close the lid.
5. Cook the eggs for 1 minute on Manual mode (high pressure).
6. Then make a quick pressure release and transfer the eggs on the plate.
7. Top the eggs with bacon slices.

Nutritional info per serve: calories 95, fat 6.2, fiber 0.1, carbs 0.6, protein 8.6

Starbucks Eggs

Prep time: 10 minutes | **Cook time:** 2 minutes | **Yield:** 2 servings

Ingredients

- 4 eggs
- 2 oz cottage cheese
- 1/3 cup Cheddar cheese, shredded
- 1 teaspoon chives, chopped
- 1 cup of water

Method

1. Crack the eggs in the bowl and mix them with chives.
2. Whisk the eggs and add shredded Cheddar cheese and cottage cheese. Stir well.
3. Then pour the eggs in the muffin molds.
4. Pour water in the instant pot and insert the steamer rack.
5. Place the eggs on the rack and cook them for 2 minutes on Manual mode (high pressure).
6. Make a quick pressure release and remove the eggs from the molds.

Nutritional info per serve: calories 227, fat 15.5, fiber 0, carbs 2, protein 19.7

Frittata with Greens

Prep time: 10 minutes | **Cook time:** 10 minutes | **Yield:** 2 servings

Ingredients

- 2 eggs, beaten
- ¼ cup heavy cream
- ½ teaspoon white pepper
- 1 tablespoon chives, chopped
- 1 teaspoon ground
- paprika
- 1 teaspoon butter, softened
- 1 tablespoon scallions, chopped
- 1 cup water, for cooking

Method

1. In the mixing bowl, mix up eggs, heavy cream, white pepper, chives, ground paprika, and scallions.
2. Then grease the frittata ramekin with softened butter.
3. Pour the egg mixture in the prepared ramekin and place it on the trivet.
4. Then pour water in the instant pot and insert the trivet inside.
5. Cook the frittata for 10 minutes on Manual mode (high pressure).
6. Then make a quick pressure release and cut the meal into halves.

Nutritional info per serve: calories 137, fat 12, fiber 0.7, carbs 2, protein 6.2

Egg Cups

Prep time: 15 minutes | **Cook time:** 13 minutes | **Yield:** 4 servings

Ingredients

- 4 eggs
- ¼ cups spinach, chopped
- ½ teaspoon chili flakes
- 2 oz Mozzarella, sliced
- 1 teaspoon butter, melted
- 1 cup water, for cooking

Method

1. Brush the muffin molds with butter.

2. Then crack the egg in every mold and sprinkle them with chili flakes and spinach.

3. Top the eggs with sliced Mozzarella.

4. Pour water and insert the steamer rack in the instant pot.

5. Put the egg cups on the rack and close the lid.

6. Cook the meal on manual mode (high pressure) for 3 minutes. Make a quick pressure release.

7. Let the cooked egg cups cool to room temperature. Remove the eggs from the muffin molds.

   Nutritional info per serve: calories 112, fat 7.8, fiber 0, carbs 0.9, protein 9.6

Noatmeal

Prep time: 10 minutes | **Cook time:** 5 hours | **Yield:** 4 servings

Ingredients

- ½ cup coconut shred
- 1 teaspoon ground cinnamon
- 1 teaspoon Erythritol
- 3 tablespoons flaxseeds
- 3 tablespoons sunflower seeds
- ½ cup coconut cream
- ½ cup of water
- ½ teaspoon butter

Method

1. In the mixing bowl, mix up coconut shred, ground cinnamon, Erythritol, flaxseeds, sunflower seeds, coconut cream, water, and butter.

2. Transfer the mixture in the instant pot bowl.

3. Set the slow cook mode and cook the meal for 5 hours.

4. Then stir it well and transfer in the serving ramekins.

   Nutritional info per serve: calories 215, fat 20.4, fiber 4.6, carbs 8.1, protein 2.1

Bacon and Cheese Bites

Prep time: 15 minutes | **Cook time:** 3 minutes | **Yield:** 2 servings

Ingredients

- 2 tablespoons coconut flour
- ½ cup Cheddar cheese, shredded
- 2 teaspoons coconut cream
- 2 bacon slices, cooked
- ½ teaspoon dried parsley
- 1 cup water, for cooking

Method

1. In the mixing bowl, mix up coconut flour, Cheddar cheese, coconut cream, and dried parsley.

2. Then chop the cooked bacon and add it in the mixture.

3. Stir it well.

4. Pour water and insert the trivet in the instant pot.

5. Line the trivet with baking paper.

6. After this, make the small balls (bites) from the cheese mixture and put them on the prepared trivet.

7. Cook the meal for 3 minutes on manual mode (high pressure).

8. Then make a quick pressure release and cool the cooked meal well.

   Nutritional info per serve: calories 258, fat 19.2, fiber 3.1, carbs 5.9, protein 15.2

Morning Burritos

Prep time: 10 minutes | Cook time: 15 minutes | Yield: 4 servings

Ingredients

- 4 keto tortillas
- 1 cup ground beef
- ¼ cup crushed tomatoes
- 1 teaspoon olive oil
- 3 oz scallions, diced
- ½ teaspoon dried cilantro

Method

1. In the mixing bowl mix up ground beef, crushed tomatoes, olive oil, scallions, and dried cilantro.

2. Put the meat mixture in the instant pot.

3. Close and seal the lid.

4. Cook the beef mixture for 15 minutes on Manual mode (high pressure).

5. Then make a quick pressure release and stir the meat well.

6. Fill the tortillas with the cooked mixture and roll them in the shape of burritos.

   Nutritional info per serve: calories 238, fat 13.3, fiber 5.1, carbs 10.8, protein 19.3

Breakfast Sandwich

Prep time: 10 minutes | **Cook time:** 15 minutes | **Yield:** 4 servings

Ingredients

- 1 cup lettuce
- 2 cups ground chicken
- 1 tablespoon coconut flour
- 1 teaspoon salt
- 1 tablespoon butter
- ½ teaspoon ground nutmeg
- 3 oz scallions, chopped

Method

1. Preheat the instant pot on saute mode for 5 minutes.
2. Then add butter and melt it.
3. Add chopped scallions
4. After this, add ground chicken and ground nutmeg. Stir the mixture well and cook for 4 minutes.
5. Then add coconut flour and salt. Saute the meal for 10 minutes.
6. Fill the lettuce with the ground chicken and transfer it on the plate. The sandwiches are cooked.

Nutritional info per serve: calories 177, fat 8.6, fiber 1.5, carbs 3.2, protein 21.1

White Cabbage Hash Browns

Prep time: 10 minutes | **Cook time:** 10 minutes | **Yield:** 3 servings

Ingredients

- 1 cup white cabbage, shredded
- 3 eggs, beaten
- ½ teaspoon ground nutmeg
- ½ teaspoon salt
- 1 tablespoon coconut oil
- ½ teaspoon onion powder
- ½ zucchini, grated

Method

1. In the mixing bowl, mix up shredded cabbage, eggs, ground nutmeg, salt, onion powder, and grated zucchini.
2. Then heat up coconut oil in the instant pot on Saute mode.
3. Make the medium hash browns from the cabbage mixture (use the tablespoon for this step).
4. After this, place the hash browns in the hot coconut oil.
5. Cook them on saute mode for 4 minutes from each side.

Nutritional info per serve: calories 116, fat 9.1, fiber 1, carbs 3.3, protein 6.3

Giant Vanilla Pancake

Prep time: 15 minutes | **Cook time:** 50 minutes | **Yield:** 6 servings

Ingredients

- ½ cup coconut flour
- 3 tablespoons swerve
- ¼ cup heavy cream
- 3 eggs, beaten
- 1 teaspoon vanilla
- extract
- ¼ cup almond flour
- 1 teaspoon baking powder
- Cooking spray

Method

1. In the mixing bowl, mix up coconut flour, swerve, heavy cream, eggs, vanilla extract, and almond flour.
2. Then add baking powder and whisk the mixture until smooth.
3. Pour the pancake mixture in the instant pot.
4. Cook the meal on manual mode (low pressure) for 50 minutes.

Nutritional info per serve: calories 122, fat 7.3, fiber 4.5, carbs 9.5, protein 5.2

Meat Cups

Prep time: 15 minutes | **Cook time:** 15 minutes | **Yield:** 4 servings

Ingredients

- 4 quill eggs
- 10 oz ground pork
- 1 jalapeno pepper, chopped
- ½ teaspoon salt
- 1 teaspoon dried dill
- 1 tablespoon butter, softened
- 1 cup water, for cooking

Method

1. In the mixing bowl, mix up ground pork, chopped jalapeno pepper, salt, dill, and butter.
2. When the meat mixture is homogenous, transfer it in the silicone muffin molds and press the surface gently.
3. Then pour water in the instant pot and insert the trivet.
4. Place the meat cups on the trivet.
5. Then crack the eggs over the meat mixture and close the lid.
6. Cook the meal on manual mode (high pressure) for 15 minutes.
7. Then make a quick pressure release.

Nutritional info per serve: calories 143, fat 6.4, fiber 0.1, carbs 0.4, protein 19.9

Bell Peppers with Omelet

Prep time: 10 minutes | **Cook time:** 14 minutes | **Yield:** 2 servings

Ingredients

- 1 large bell pepper
- 2 eggs, beaten
- 1 tablespoon coconut cream
- ¼ teaspoon salt
- ¼ teaspoon dried oregano
- 1 cup of water

Method

1. Cut the bell peppers into halves and remove the seeds.
2. After this, in the mixing bowl mix up eggs, coconut cream, salt, and oregano.
3. Pour water in the instant pot and insert the rack.
4. Then pour the egg mixture in the pepper halves.
5. Transfer the peppers on the rack and close the lid.
6. Cook the meal on Manual mode (high pressure) for 14 minutes. Then make a quick pressure release.

Nutritional info per serve: calories 100, fat 6.3, fiber 1.1, carbs 5.4, protein 6.3

Stuffed Hard-Boiled Eggs

Prep time: 10 minutes | **Cook time:** 5 minutes | **Yield:** 6 servings

Ingredients

- 6 eggs
- 3 oz Provolone cheese, grated
- 1 teaspoon chili pepper, chopped
- 1 tablespoon coconut cream
- ½ teaspoon ground paprika
- 1 cup of water

Method

1. Pour water in the instant pot.
2. Add eggs and close the lid.
3. Cook the on manual mode (high pressure) for 5 minutes. Then allow the natural pressure release and open the lid.
4. Cool and peel the eggs.
5. After this, cut the eggs into halves and remove the egg yolks.
6. Mash the egg yolks and mix them up with grated cheese, coconut cream, chili pepper, and ground paprika.
7. Then fill the egg white halves with egg yolk mixture.

Nutritional info per serve: calories 119, fat 8.8, fiber 0.2, carbs 1, protein 9.3

Bacon Avocado Bomb

Prep time: 10 minutes | **Cook time:** 25 minutes | **Yield:** 4 servings

Ingredients

- 1 avocado, pilled, pitted, halved
- 4 bacon slices
- ½ teaspoon ground cinnamon
- 1 teaspoon coconut cream
- ½ teaspoon chili flakes

Method

1. Sprinkle the avocado with ground cinnamon and chili flakes.
2. Then fill it with coconut cream and wrap in the bacon slices.
3. Secure the avocado bomb with toothpicks, if needed and wrap in the foil.
4. Place it in the instant pot and close the lid.
5. Cook the bomb on saute mode for 25 minutes.
6. Then remove the foil and slice the avocado bomb into the servings.

Nutritional info per serve: calories 209, fat 18, fiber 3.6, carbs 4.9, protein 8

Swedish Meatballs

Prep time: 15 minutes | **Cook time:** 25 minutes | **Yield:** 2 servings

Ingredients

- 1/3 cup ground beef
- ¼ cup ground pork
- ¼ teaspoon white pepper
- 1 teaspoon avocado oil
- ½ teaspoon ground black pepper
- 1 teaspoon coconut flour
- ¼ teaspoon Erythritol
- ½ cup coconut cream

Method

1. In the mixing bowl, mix up ground beef, ground pork, white pepper, ground black pepper, and Erythritol.
2. Make the small meatballs.
3. Preheat the instant pot on saute mode for 2 minutes and add avocado oil.
4. Put the meatballs in the hot oil in one layer and cook them for 3 minutes from each side.
5. Meanwhile, mix up coconut cream and coconut flour.
6. Pour the liquid over the meatballs and close the lid. Cook the meal on saute mode for 15 minutes.

Nutritional info per serve: calories 331, fat 26.5, fiber 4, carbs 8.3, protein 16.8

Cheese Roll-Ups

Prep time: 10 minutes | **Cook time:** 5 minutes | **Yield:** 3 servings

Ingredients

- 3 turkey lunch meat slices
- 3 oz Parmesan, grated
- ½ teaspoon minced garlic
- 1 tablespoon cream cheese
- ½ teaspoon olive oil

Method

1. Heat up the olive oil on saute mode.
2. Then place the turkey slices in the hot oil and cook them for 2 minutes from each side.
3. Meanwhile, in the mixing bowl mix up cream cheese, minced garlic, and Parmesan.
4. Transfer the cooked turkey slices on the plate and spread them with cheese mixture.
5. Roll up the turkey slices and secure them with the toothpicks.

Nutritional info per serve: calories 160, fat 8, fiber 0, carbs5 1.3, protein 21.4

Breakfast Taco Skillet

Prep time: 10 minutes | **Cook time:** 17 minutes | **Yield:** 6 servings

Ingredients

- ½ avocado, chopped
- 3 jalapeno peppers, chopped
- 2 cups ground beef
- 1 teaspoon chili flakes
- 1/3 cup coconut milk
- ¾ cup black olives, sliced
- 1 teaspoon coconut oil
- 2 eggs, beaten

Method

1. Melt the coconut oil on saute mode for 2 minutes.
2. Then add ground beef and chili flakes.
3. Cook the meat on saute mode for 4 minutes. Stir it well.
4. Add jalapeno peppers, coconut milk, olives, and eggs,
5. Stir the mixture until homogenous.
6. Add chopped avocado and close the lid.
7. Cook the meal on manual mode (high pressure) for 10 minutes. Then ake the quick pressure release.

Nutritional info per serve: calories 201, fat 16, fiber 2.2, carbs 3.9, protein 11.4

Meat and Cauliflower Bake

Prep time: 10 minutes | **Cook time:** 15 minutes | **Yield:** 4 servings

Ingredients

- 4 eggs, beaten
- 1 cup cauliflower, shredded
- ½ cup ground chicken
- 1 tablespoon Italian seasonings
- ½ teaspoon salt
- ¼ cup Cheddar cheese, shredded
- 1 cup water, for cooking

Method

1. In the mixing bowl, mix up beaten eggs, shredded cauliflower, Italian seasonings, and salt.
2. Then pour the mixture in 4 ramekins.
3. Add ground chicken.
4. Top the ramekins with Cheddar cheese.
5. Then pour the water in the instant pot, insert the trivet.
6. Put the ramekins on the trivet and close the lid.
7. Cook the meal on manual mode (high pressure) for 15 minutes. Then make a quick pressure release.

Nutritional info per serve: calories 142, fat 9.1, fiber 0.6, carbs 2.1, protein 12.9

Pulled Pork Hash with Eggs

Prep time: 10 minutes | **Cook time:** 15 minutes | **Yield:** 4 servings

Ingredients

- 4 eggs
- 10 oz pulled pork, shredded
- 1 teaspoon coconut oil
- 1 teaspoon red
- pepper
- 1 teaspoon fresh cilantro, chopped
- 1 tomato, chopped
- ¼ cup of water

Method

1. Melt the coconut oil in the instant pot on saute mode.
2. Then add pulled pork, red pepper, cilantro, water, and chopped tomato.
3. Cook the ingredients for 5 minutes.
4. Then stir it well with the help of the spatula and crack the eggs over it.
5. Close the lid.
6. Cook the meal on manual mode (high pressure) for 7 minutes. Then make a quick pressure release.

Nutritional info per serve: calories 275, fat 18.3, fiber 0.6, carbs 5.7, protein 22.4

Kale and Eggs Bake

Prep time: 10 minutes | **Cook time:** 10 minutes | **Yield:** 2 servings

Ingredients

- ½ cup kale, chopped
- 3 eggs, beaten
- 1 tablespoon organic almond milk
- 1 teaspoon coconut
- oil, melted
- ¼ teaspoon ground black pepper
- 1 cup water, for cooking

Method

1. In the mixing bowl, mix up chopped kale, eggs, almond milk, and ground black pepper.

2. Grease the ramekins with coconut oil.

3. Pour the kale-egg mixture in the ramekins and flatten it with the help of the spatula, if needed.

4. Pour water and insert the trivet in the instant pot.

5. Put the ramekins with egg mixture on the trivet and close the lid.

6. Cook the breakfast on manual mode (high pressure) for 10 minutes. Make a quick pressure release.

Nutritional info per serve: calories 126, fat 9.1, fiber 0.3, carbs 2.6, protein 8.9

Egg Cups on the Run

Prep time: 10 minutes | **Cook time:** 6 minutes | **Yield:** 3 servings

Ingredients

- 3 eggs, beaten
- 1 oz tomato, chopped
- 1 oz celery stalk, chopped
- 1 tablespoon chives, chopped
- 3 oz Cheddar cheese, shredded
- ½ cup heavy cream
- ¼ teaspoon chili powder
- 1 cup water, for cooking

Method

1. In the mixing bowl, mix up eggs, tomato, celery stalk, chives, cheese, heavy cream, and chili powder.

2. Then pour the mixture in the glass cups.

3. Pour water and insert the steamer rack in the instant pot.

4. Then place the glass cups with egg mixture on the rack. Close and seal the lid.

5. Cook the meal on manual (high pressure) for 6 minutes. Make a quick pressure release.

Nutritional info per serve: calories 250, fat 21.3, fiber 0.4, carbs 2.1, protein 13.2

Margherita Egg Cups

Prep time: 10 minutes | **Cook time:** 5 minutes | **Yield:** 2 servings

Ingredients

- 2 eggs
- 4 oz Mozzarella, shredded
- ½ tomato, chopped
- 1 teaspoon butter,
- softened
- ½ teaspoon fresh basil, chopped
- 1 cup water, for cooking

Method

1. Grease the small ramekins with softened butter and crack the eggs inside.

2. Then top the eggs with chopped tomato, basil, and Mozzarella.

3. Pour water and insert the steamer rack in the instant pot.

4. Place the ramekins with eggs on the rack. Close and seal the lid.

5. Cook the meal on manual (high pressure) for 5 minutes. Allow the natural pressure release for 5 minutes.

Nutritional info per serve: calories 243, fat 16.3, fiber 0.2, carbs 3, protein 21.7

Chicken Strips

Prep time: 10 minutes | **Cook time:** 15 minutes | **Yield:** 5 servings

Ingredients

- 1-pound chicken fillet
- ½ teaspoon ground turmeric
- ½ teaspoon salt
- ½ teaspoon ground
- black pepper
- 2 tablespoons heavy cream
- 1 cup of coconut milk
- 1 teaspoon olive oil

Method

1. Cut the chicken fillet into the strips and sprinkle with ground turmeric, salt, ground black pepper, and heavy cream.

2. Preheat the olive oil on saute mode for 3 minutes,

3. Then place the chicken strips in hot oil in one layer. Cook them for 1 minute from each side and add coconut cream.

4. Close and seal the lid.

5. Cook the chicken strips on Manual (high pressure) for 10 minutes. Make a quick pressure release.

Nutritional info per serve: calories 313, fat 21.3, fiber 1.2, carbs 3.1, protein 27.5

Nut Yogurt

Prep time: 10 minutes | **Cook time:** 6 minutes | **Yield:** 3 servings

Ingredients

- 1 cup of coconut yogurt
- ½ oz pistachio nuts, chopped
- ½ oz hazelnuts, chopped
- ½ oz macadamia nuts, chopped
- 1 teaspoon Erythritol
- ½ teaspoon coconut oil

Method

1. Preheat the coconut oil on saute mode for 1 minute.

2. When the oil is hot, add pistachio nuts, hazelnuts, and macadamia nuts. Cook them on saute mode for 5 minutes. Stir the nuts constantly.

3. Then cool the buts well and mix them up with Erythritol and coconut yogurt.

4. Put the cooked meal in the serving jars.

    Nutritional info per serve: calories 132, fat 10.7, fiber 1.3, carbs 8.9, protein 3.3

Bacon Casserole

Prep time: 10 minutes | **Cook time:** 10 minutes | **Yield:** 6 servings

Ingredients

- 4 bacon slices, chopped
- 1 teaspoon olive oil
- 6 eggs, beaten
- ½ cup spinach, chopped
- ½ cup heavy cream
- 1 teaspoon chili flakes
- 3 oz Parmesan, grated
- 1 teaspoon ground paprika
- 1 cup water, for cooking

Method

1. Preheat the instant pot on Saute mode for 2-3 minutes.

2. Then put the chopped bacon inside and cook it on saute mode for 5 minutes or until it is crunchy.

3. Then transfer the cooked bacon in the mixing bowl. Add the eggs, spinach, heavy cream, chili flakes, paprika, and Parmesan. Carefully stir the. Clean the instant pot and pour water and insert the steamer rack inside.

4. After this, pour the mixture in the baking mold/ramekin and cover with foil. Cook the casserole on manual (high pressure) for 15 minutes. Allow the natural pressure release for 10 minutes.

    Nutritional info per serve: calories 220, fat 17.2, fiber 0.2, carbs 1.6, protein 15.1

Feta Stuffed Chicken

Prep time: 15 minutes | **Cook time:** 17 minutes | **Yield:** 5 servings

Ingredients

- 1-pound chicken breast, skinless, boneless
- 1 tablespoon Italian seasonings
- 1 teaspoon olive oil
- 3 oz Feta cheese, crumbled
- 1 cup water, for cooking

Method

1. Beat the chicken breast gently with the help of the kitchen hammer.

2. Then make a cut in the breast (to get the pocket).

3. Rub the chicken with Italian seasonings and olive oil.

4. Then fill the "chicken pocket" with crumbled Feta.

5. After this, wrap the chicken breast in the foil.

6. Pour water and insert the steamer rack in the instant pot.

7. Place the chicken on the rack; close and seal the lid

8. Cook the meal on manual mode (high pressure) for 17 minutes; allow the natural pressure release for 5 minutes.

    Nutritional info per serve: calories 165, fat 7.7, fiber 0, carbs 1, protein 21.7

Pancetta Eggs

Prep time: 10 minutes | **Cook time:** 5 minutes | **Yield:** 4 servings

Ingredients

- 2 oz Pancetta, fried
- 4 eggs
- 1 teaspoon chives, chopped
- ½ teaspoon salt
- Cooking spray
- 1 cup water, for cooking

Method

1. Spray the egg molds with cooking spray.

2. Crack the eggs in the egg molds and sprinkle with salt, chives, and Pancetta. Stir every egg mixture gently.

3. Then pour water and insert the steamer rack in the instant pot.

4. Put the egg molds in the instant pot. Close and seal the lid.

5. Cook the meal on manual mode (high pressure) for 5 minutes. Make a quick pressure release.

    Nutritional info per serve: calories 140, fat 10.3, fiber 0, carbs 0.6, protein 10.8

Cupcake Mugs

Prep time: 20 minutes | **Cook time:** 17 minutes | **Yield:** 6 servings

Ingredients

- 4 eggs, beaten
- ½ teaspoon ground cinnamon
- ½ teaspoon vanilla extract
- 1 cup almond flour
- 1 teaspoon baking powder
- 1/3 cup coconut cream
- 2 tablespoon Erythritol
- 1 teaspoon butter, melted
- 1 cup water, for cooking

Method

1. Mix up together all ingredients and pour the mixture in the glass jars.
2. Then pour water and insert the steamer rack in the instant pot.
3. Cover every glass jar with foil and secure the edges.
4. Then place the jars on the rack. Close and seal the lid.
5. Cook the cupcake mugs on Manual (high pressure) for 17 minutes.
6. Then make a quick pressure release and let the cooked meal cool for 10 minutes before serving.

Nutritional info per serve: calories 192, fat 15.6, fiber 2.4, carbs 10.6, protein 8

Chicken Frittata

Prep time: 10 minutes | **Cook time:** 6 minutes | **Yield:** 2 servings

Ingredients

- 3 eggs, beaten
- 4 oz chicken fillet, boiled
- 1 teaspoon coconut oil
- ¼ teaspoon cayenne pepper
- 1 cup water, for cooking

Method

1. Pour water in the instant pot.
2. Then shred the boiled chicken fillet and mix it up with eggs, coconut oil, and cayenne pepper.
3. Pour the mixture in the instant pot baking mold and transfer it in the instant pot.
4. Close and seal the lid and cook the frittata on manual mode (high pressure) for 6 minutes.
5. When the time of cooking is finished, make a quick pressure release and cut the frittata into servings.

Nutritional info per serve: calories 222, fat 13.1, fiber 0.1, carbs 0.6, protein 24.7

Cauliflower Quiche

Prep time: 10 minutes | **Cook time:** 10 minutes | **Yield:** 2 servings

Ingredients

- 1 cup cauliflower, chopped
- ¼ cup Cheddar cheese, shredded
- 5 eggs, beaten
- 1 teaspoon butter
- 1 teaspoon dried oregano
- 1 cup of water

Method

1. Grease the instant pot baking pan with butter from inside.
2. Pour water in the instant pot.
3. Sprinkle the cauliflower with dried oregano and put it in the prepared baking pan. Flatten the vegetables gently.
4. After this, add eggs and stir the vegetables.
5. Top the quiche with shredded cheese and transfer it in the instant pot. Close and seal the lid.
6. Cook the quiche on manual mode (high pressure) for 10 minutes. Make a quick pressure release.

Nutritional info per serve: calories 246, fat 17.7, fiber 1.6, carbs 4.2, protein 18.5

Ham Muffins

Prep time: 10 minutes | **Cook time:** 6 minutes | **Yield:** 2 servings

Ingredients

- 2 eggs, beaten
- 4 oz ham, chopped
- ½ teaspoon avocado
- oil
- 1 cup water, for cooking

Method

1. Pour water in the instant pot.
2. Then brush the muffin molds with avocado oil from inside.
3. In the mixing bowl, mix up ham and beaten eggs.
4. After this, pour the mixture into the muffin molds.
5. Place the muffins in the instant pot. Close and seal the lid.
6. Cook the meal on manual mode (high pressure) for 6 minutes. Then make a quick pressure release and remove the muffins.

Nutritional info per serve: calories 192, fat 15.6, fiber 2.4, carbs 10.6, protein 8

Spanakopita

Prep time: 20 minutes | **Cook time:** 15 minutes | **Yield:** 4 servings

Ingredients

- ½ cup coconut flour
- 3 eggs, beaten
- 2 tablespoons goat milk butter
- 1 cup spinach, chopped
- 1 oz scallions, chopped
- 3 tablespoons cream cheese
- 4 egg whites, whisked
- 1 cup water, for cooking

Method

1. Make the dough: in the mixing bowl mix up coconut flour, eggs, and goat milk butter. Knead the dough.
2. Then place the dough in the round mold and flatten in the shape of the pie crust.
3. Pour water in the instant pot and insert the steamer rack.
4. Put the mold with the pie crust on the rack. Close and seal the lid. Cook the pie crust for 10 minutes on manual mode (high pressure) + quick pressure release.
5. After this, mix up spinach, scallions, cream cheese, and eggs,
6. Pour the mixture over the cooked pie crust.
7. Cook the spanakopita for 5 minutes more on manual mode (high pressure). Then allow the natural pressure release for 5 minutes.

Nutritional info per serve: calories 157, fat 12.3, fiber 1, carbs 2.5, protein 8.9

Chili Roasted Eggs

Prep time: 5 minutes | **Cook time:** 7 minutes | **Yield:** 3 servings

Ingredients

- 1 teaspoon coconut oil
- 3 eggs
- ½ teaspoon chili flakes

Method

1. Heat up coconut oil in the instant pot on Saute mode.
2. When the coconut oil is hot, crack the eggs in the instant pot bowl and sprinkle with chili flakes.
3. Cook the eggs on saute mode for 5 minutes.

Nutritional info per serve: calories 76, fat 5.9, fiber 0, carbs 0.4, protein 5.5

Vegetable Frittata

Prep time: 10 minutes | **Cook time:** 10 minutes | **Yield:** 4 servings

Ingredients

- 4 eggs, beaten
- 2 oz Pecorino cheese, grated
- 3 oz okra, chopped
- 2 oz radish, chopped
- 1 tablespoon cream cheese
- 1 teaspoon sesame oil

Method

1. Heat up sesame oil in the instant pot on saute mode.
2. Add chopped okra and radish and saute the vegetables for 4 minutes.
3. Then stir them well and add cream cheese and beaten eggs.
4. Stir the mixture well and top with cheese.
5. Close the lid and cook the frittata on saute mode for 6 minutes more.

Nutritional info per serve: calories 163, fat 12.1, fiber 0.9, carbs 2.5, protein 11.9

Sausage Puffs

Prep time: 15 minutes | **Cook time:** 10 minutes | **Yield:** 6 servings

Ingredients

- 9 oz ground sausages, fried
- 1 egg, beaten
- ¼ cup coconut flour
- ¼ teaspoon baking powder
- 3 oz Provolone cheese, grated
- 1 tablespoon cream cheese
- 1 cup water, for cooking

Method

1. In the mixing bowl, mix up ground sausages, egg, coconut flour, baking powder, grated Parmesan, and cream cheese.
2. Make the small puff from the ground sausages and put in the non-stick baking pan.
3. Pour water and insert the pan with sausage puffs in the instant pot.
4. Close and seal the lid.
5. Cook the meal on manual (high pressure) for 10 minutes. Make a quick pressure release.

Nutritional info per serve: calories 230, fat 17.8, fiber 1.7, carbs 3.2, protein 13.6

Spicy Eggs

Prep time: 5 minutes | **Cook time:** 3 minutes | **Yield:** 2 servings

Ingredients

- 4 eggs
- ¾ teaspoon chili powder
- ¼ teaspoon jalapeno pepper
- 1 teaspoon cream cheese

Method

1. Pour 1 cup of water in the instant pot bowl and add eggs.
2. Close the lid of the instant pot and seal it.
3. Chose the "Steam" program + High Pressure. Cook the eggs for 3 minutes. Make QPR.
4. Place the eggs in the icy water.
5. Peel the eggs and cut them into the halves.
6. Sprinkle the egg halves with the chili powder.
7. In the shallow bowl mix up cream cheese and chopped jalapeno pepper.
8. Top the eggs with jalapeno mixture.

   Nutritional info per serve: calories 135, fat 9.5, fiber 0.4, carbs 1.3, protein 11.3

Cheddar Muffins

Prep time: 10 minutes | **Cook time:** 12 minutes | **Yield:** 3 servings

Ingredients

- 2 oz Cheddar cheese, shredded
- 2 tablespoons almond flour
- 2 tablespoon butter, softened
- 1 tablespoon heavy cream
- ¼ teaspoon baking powder
- ½ teaspoon lemon juice
- 1 cup water, for cooking

Method

1. Pour water in the instant pot.
2. Then mix up together all remaining ingredients and stir until homogenous.
3. Put the muffin batter in the muffin molds and insert them in the instant pot.
4. Close and seal the lid.
5. Cook the Cheddar muffins for 12 minutes on high pressure (manual mode).
6. When the time is finished, make a quick pressure release.

   Nutritional info per serve: calories 269, fat 25.1, fiber 2, carbs 4.6, protein 8.9

Mushroom Toast

Prep time: 10 minutes | **Cook time:** 12 minutes | **Yield:** 3 servings

Ingredients

- 1 cup mushrooms, grinded
- 2 eggs, beaten
- 2 tablespoons coconut flour
- 1 tablespoon chives, chopped
- 1 tablespoon butter

Method

1. In the mixing bowl, mix up grinded mushrooms, eggs, coconut flour, and chives.
2. Stir the mixture with the help of the spoon until it is homogenous.
3. Then melt butter in the instant pot on saute mode.
4. With the help of the spoon make the medium size toasts from the mushroom mixture and place them in the hot butter.
5. Saute the toasts for 5 minutes from each side.

   Nutritional info per serve: calories 121, fat 8.2 fiber 3.6, carbs 6.4, protein 5.8

Morning Aromatic Casserole

Prep time: 7 minutes | **Cook time:** 9 minutes | **Yield:** 3 servings

Ingredients

- 3 eggs, beaten
- ¼ cup coconut cream
- ¼ teaspoon salt
- 3 oz Brussel sprouts, chopped
- 2 oz tomato, chopped
- 3 oz provolone cheese, shredded
- 1 teaspoon butter
- 1 teaspoon smoked paprika

Method

1. Grease the instant pot pan with the butter.
2. Put eggs in the bowl, add salt, and smoked paprika. Whisk the eggs well.
3. After this, add chopped Brussel sprouts and tomato.
4. Pour the mixture into the instant pot pan and sprinkle over with the shredded cheese.
5. Pour 1 cup of the water in the instant pot. Then place the pan with the egg mixture and close the lid.
6. Cook the meal on "Manual" (High pressure) for 4 minutes.
7. Then make naturally release for 5 minutes.

   Nutritional info per serve: calories 237, fat 18.2, fiber 2, carbs 5.8, protein 14.5

Cups with Greens

Prep time: 6 minutes | **Cook time:** 3 minutes | **Yield:** 2 servings

Ingredients

- 3 eggs, beaten
- ¼ cup cauliflower stalks, chopped
- 2 oz broccoli raab, chopped
- 1 tablespoon heavy cream
- ½ teaspoon ground black pepper
- ¾ teaspoon butter

Method

1. Blend the cauliflower stalk and broccoli raab in the blender until smooth.
2. Mix up together the blended greens and beaten eggs.
3. Add heavy cream, ground black pepper, and butter.
4. Pour the water in the instant pot.
5. After this, pour the egg mixture into the small cups and transfer them in the instant pot.
6. Close the lid and cook on the "Manual" program (High Pressure). Cook the meal for 3 minutes. Make a quick release.

Nutritional info per serve: calories 143, fat 10.8, fiber 0.4, carbs 2.6, protein 9.4

Kale Omelet

Prep time: 5 minutes | **Cook time:** 10 minutes | **Yield:** 2 servings

Ingredients

- 2 eggs
- 1 cup kale, chopped
- 1 teaspoon heavy cream
- 2/3 teaspoon white pepper
- ½ teaspoon butter

Method

1. Grease the instant pot pan with butter.
2. Beat the eggs in the separated bowl and whisk them well.
3. After this, add heavy cream and white pepper. Stir it gently.
4. Place the chopped kale in the greased pan and add the whisked eggs.
5. Pour 1 cup of water in the instant pot.
6. Place the trivet in the instant pot and transfer the egg mixture pan on the trivet.
7. Close the instant pot and set the "Manual" (High Pressure) program and cook the frittata for 5 minutes. NPR for 5 minutes.

Nutritional info per serve: calories 98, fat 6.3, fiber 0.7, carbs 4.4, protein 6.7

Cheese Jalapenos

Prep time: 10 minutes | **Cook time:** 5 minutes | **Yield:** 2 servings

Ingredients

- 2 jalapeno pepper
- 2 oz Provolone cheese, grated
- 1 egg, beaten
- ½ teaspoon ground paprika
- 1 cup of water

Method

1. In the mixing bowl, mix up cheese, eggs, and ground paprika.
2. Then cut the jalapeno peppers into halves and remove the seeds.
3. Fill the peppers with cheese mixture.
4. Pour water in the instant pot. Insert the trivet.
5. Place the jalapenos on the trivet. Close and seal the lid.
6. Cook the meal on manual mode (high pressure) for 5 minutes. Then make quick pressure release.

Nutritional info per serve: calories 137, fat 9.9, fiber 0.6, carbs 1.9, protein 10.3

Zucchini Roll

Prep time: 8 minutes | **Cook time:** 12 minutes | **Yield:** 2 servings

Ingredients

- ½ zucchini, grated
- 9 oz chicken breast, skinless, boneless
- 1 tablespoon butter
- ½ teaspoon white pepper
- ¼ teaspoon thyme

Method

1. Beat the chicken breast well with the help of the kitchen hammer to get the tender piece.
2. Then sprinkle the chicken breast with the white pepper and thyme.
3. Put the grated zucchini over the chicken breast and flatten it well.
4. Roll up the chicken breast.
5. Wrap the zucchini roll in the foil.
6. Set the instant pot mode "Poultry" and place the zucchini roll in the instant pot bowl.
7. Cook the zucchini roll for 12 minutes. Then make naturally pressure release.
8. Slice the cooked zucchini roll.

Nutritional info per serve: calories 206, fat 9.1, fiber 0.7, carbs 2.1, protein 27.8

Quail Egg Bites

Prep time: 5 minutes | **Cook time:** 7 minutes | **Yield:** 2 servings

Ingredients

- 6 quail eggs, beaten grated
- 1 oz Swiss cheese, - ½ teaspoon butter

Method

1. Grease the instant pot pan with the butter generously.
2. Then beat the eggs in the bowl and whisk well.
3. Add cheese.
4. Stir the quail eggs gently and transfer into the greased instant pot pan.
5. Place the pan into the instant pot and close the lid.
6. Cook the meal on "Manual" mode (High pressure - QPR) for 4 minutes to get the solid eggs.
7. Cut the cooked quail mixture into bars.

Nutritional info per serve: calories 105, fat 7.9, fiber 0, carbs 0.9, protein 7.4

Breakfast Muffins

Prep time: 5 minutes | **Cook time:** 15 minutes | **Yield:** 2 servings

Ingredients

- 2 eggs, beaten - 2 tablespoons almond flour
- ¼ cup organic almond milk - ¾ teaspoon butter

Method

1. Pour 1 cup of water in the instant pot bowl.
2. Beat the eggs in the bowl and combine together with the almond milk and almond flour.
3. Whisk the mixture.
4. Put the egg mixture in the muffin molds. Add butter.
5. Place the trivet in the instant pot and transfer the muffins in it.
6. Close the instant pot lid and set the "Steam".
7. Cook the muffins for 10 minutes.
8. After this, make the quick release (QPR) for 5 minutes.

Nutritional info per serve: calories 256, fat 21.3, fiber 3, carbs 6.3, protein 12.1

Egg Pate

Prep time: 10 minutes | **Cook time:** 5 minutes | **Yield:** 6 servings

Ingredients

- 8 eggs cheese
- 1 oz avocado, mashed - ½ teaspoon salt
- 2 tablespoons cream - 1 cup water, for cooking

Method

1. Pour 1 cup of water in the instant pot bowl and add eggs.
2. Set the "Steam" mode on your instant pot and cook the eggs for 5 minutes (QR).
3. Meanwhile, mix up cream cheese and mashed avocado.
4. Peel the cooked eggs and put them in the blender. Blend the eggs until smooth.
5. Churn together eggs and avocado mash mixture.
6. The egg pate is cooked.

Nutritional info per serve: calories 105, fat 7.9, fiber 0.3, carbs 1, protein 7.7

Bacon Kebob

Prep time: 7 minutes | **Cook time:** 10 minutes | **Yield:** 2 servings

Ingredients

- 1 eggplant oil
- 4 bacon slices - ½ teaspoon ground black pepper
- 1 tablespoon coconut

Method

1. Chop the eggplant into the cubes and sprinkle with the coconut oil and ground black pepper.
2. Wrap the vegetables with bacon and string on the wooden skewers.
3. Place the kebobs on the trivet and transfer the trivet in the instant pot.
4. Add ½ cup of water in the instant pot bowl and close the lid.
5. Cook the meal on "Manual" (High Pressure) mode for 8 minutes. Then make naturally pressure release for 5 minutes.

Nutritional info per serve: calories 323, fat 23.1, fiber 8.2, carbs 14.4, protein 16.4

Lemon Fish Cakes

Prep time: 15 minutes | **Cook time:** 6 minutes | **Yield:** 2 servings

Ingredients

- 1 teaspoon butter
- ½ teaspoon dried thyme
- ¾ teaspoon garlic

  powder
- 10 oz salmon cod fillet
- 1 oz lemon, sliced

Method

1. Grind the cod fillet and mix it up with the garlic powder and dried thyme.

2. Blend the lemon and add it to the fish mixture.

3. Grease the instant pot pan with the butter.

4. Make the fish cakes from the mixture and put it in the instant pot.

5. Cook them on saute mode for 3 minutes from each side or until they are light brown.

   Nutritional info per serve: calories 286, fat 18.2, fiber 1.4, carbs 4.3, protein 28.6

Egg&Cheese

Prep time: 10 minutes | **Cook time:** 6 minutes | **Yield:** 1 serving

Ingredients

- 2 eggs, beaten
- 1 oz Parmesan, grated
- 1 oz Swiss cheese, grated
- ¼ cup heavy cream
- ½ teaspoon dried cilantro
- ½ teaspoon almond butter

Method

1. Toss the almond butter in the instant pot and melt it on saute mode.

2. Then add eggs and cream cheese. Sprinkle the ingredients with dried cilantro and cook on saute mode for 4 minutes.

3. When the egg mixture is solid, stir it gently to get the small egg pieces.

4. After this, add grated cheese and close the lid. Cook the meal for 2 minutes more.

   Nutritional info per serve: calories 192, fat 15.6, fiber 2.4, carbs 10.6, protein 8

Omelet "3-Cheese"

Prep time: 5 minutes | **Cook time:** 3 minutes | **Yield:** 2 servings

Ingredients

- 2 eggs, beaten
- 1 oz Mozzarella, shredded
- ¾ teaspoon dried oregano
- ½ teaspoon coconut oil
- 1 oz Cheddar cheese, shredded
- 1 oz Provolone cheese, grated
- ½ cup water, for cooking

Method

1. Mix up eggs, all cheese, and dried oregano.

2. After this, grease the pan with the coconut and pour the egg mixture inside.

3. Pour ½ cup of water in the instant pot bowl and place the pan with eggs inside.

4. Cook omelet on "Manual" mode for 4 minutes (natural pressure release).

   Nutritional info per serve: calories 221, fat 16.5, fiber 0.2, carbs 1.7, protein 16.8

Cream Shrimps

Prep time: 5 minutes | **Cook time:** 5 minutes | **Yield:** 2 servings

Ingredients

- 8 oz shrimps, peeled
- ½ cup heavy cream
- 1 teaspoon butter
- ½ teaspoon chili flakes

Method

1. Set the "Meat/Stew" mode on the instant pot

2. Toss butter in the instant pot bowl and add shrimps.

3. Add all remaining ingredients and close the lid.

4. Cook the shrimps for 5 minutes on the "Meat/Stew" mode.

   Nutritional info per serve: calories 255, fat 14.9, fiber 0, carbs 2.6, protein 26.5

Breakfast Mash

Prep time: 5 minutes | **Cook time:** 7 minutes | **Yield:** 2 servings

Ingredients

- ¾ cup shredded coconut
- 2 tablespoons coconut flour
- ½ cup of coconut milk
- 1 teaspoon ground flax meal
- 1 tablespoon Erythritol
- 1 teaspoon vanilla extract

Method

1. Mix up together all ingredients and transfer in the instant pot.

2. Cook the mash on saute mode for 7 minutes. Stir it constantly.

3. The meal is cooked when it starts to boil.

   Nutritional info per serve: calories 285, fat 25.3, fiber 7.2, carbs 13.7, protein 3.5

3-Cheese Quiche Cups

Prep time: 10 minutes | **Cook time:** 6 minutes | **Yield:** 6 servings

Ingredients

- 6 eggs, beaten
- 2 tablespoon cream cheese
- 1 teaspoon Italian seasonings
- ¼ cup Cheddar cheese, shredded
- 3 oz Monterey Jack cheese, shredded
- 2 oz Mozzarella, shredded
- 1 cup water, for cooking

Method

1. Pour water in the instant pot.

2. In the mixing bowl, mix up eggs cream cheese, Italian seasonings, and all types of cheese.

3. Pour the mixture in the baking cups (molds) and place them in the instant pot.

4. Close and seal the lid.

5. Cook the quiche cups for 6 minutes on manual mode (high pressure).

6. Make a quick pressure release.

   Nutritional info per serve: calories 175, fat 13.3, fiber 1, carbs 1, protein 13.1

Stuffed Lettuce Boats

Prep time: 10 minutes | **Cook time:** 5 minutes | **Yield:** 2 servings

Ingredients

- 4 oz shrimps
- 1 tablespoon heavy cream
- ¾ teaspoon salt
- ¼ teaspoon dried oregano
- 4 lettuce leaves
- ½ teaspoon butter

Method

1. Peel the shrimps sprinkle with the salt, heavy cream, and dried oregano.

2. Chop the garlic clove and add in shrimps.

3. Set the "Stew" mode and put the shrimp mixture inside. Cook the meal for 5 minutes.

4. Fill the lettuce leaves with cooked shrimps.

   Nutritional info per serve: calories 104, fat 4.7, fiber 0.1, carbs 1.5, protein 13.1

Sides & Appetizers

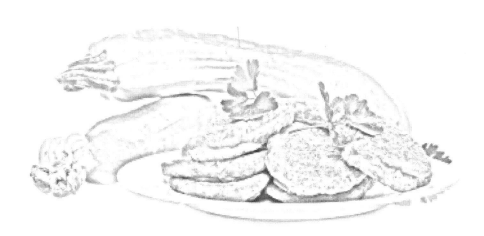

Cauliflower Queso

Prep time: 10 minutes | **Cook time:** 30 minutes | **Yield:** 5 servings

Ingredients

- 2 cups cauliflower, chopped
- 1/3 cup cream cheese
- ½ cup Cheddar cheese
- 1 jalapeno, chopped
- 2 oz scallions, diced
- 1 tablespoon nutritional yeast
- 1 tablespoon olive oil
- 2 garlic cloves, diced

Method

1. Put chopped cauliflower, cream cheese, Cheddar cheese, jalapeno, diced scallions, nutritional yeast, olive oil, and diced garlic clove.

2. Stir the mixture well with the help of the spoon and close the lid.

3. Cook the queso for 30 minutes on saute mode. Stir meal every 5 minutes to avoid burning.

Nutritional info per serve: calories 146, fat 12.1, fiber 1.9, carbs 5, protein 6

Jalapenos with Cheese

Prep time: 10 minutes | **Cook time:** 7 minutes | **Yield:** 4 servings

Ingredients

- 4 jalapeno peppers
- 1 egg, beaten
- ½ cup Monterey Jack cheese, shredded
- 1 teaspoon almond butter, softened
- 1 cup water, for cooking

Method

1. Cut the jalapenos into halves and remove the seeds.

2. In the mixing bowl, mix up softened almond butter, cheese, and egg.

3. Then fill the jalapeno halves with cheese mixture.

4. Put the jalapenos in the ramekin.

5. Then pour water and insert the rack in the instant pot.

6. Put the ramekin with jalapenos on the rack and close the lid.

7. Cook the meal for 7 minutes on manual (high pressure). Make a quick pressure release.

Nutritional info per serve: calories 99, fat 7.8, fiber 1, carbs 2, protein 5.9

Sweet Smokies

Prep time: 5 minutes | **Cook time:** 15 minutes | **Yield:** 3 servings

Ingredients

- 1 teaspoon Erythritol
- ½ teaspoon sesame seeds
- 2 tablespoons keto BBQ sauce
- 8 oz cocktail sausages
- 1/3 cup chicken broth

Method

1. Put Erythritol, sesame seeds, BBQ sauce, and chicken broth in the instant pot.

2. Preheat the mixture on saute mode for 2 minutes.

3. Then add cocktail sausages and stir the mixture well.

4. Cook the meal for 10 minutes on saute mode. Stir the sausages every 2 minutes.

Nutritional info per serve: calories 49, fat 2.5, fiber 5.7, carbs 0.1, protein 2.3

Bacon Deviled Eggs

Prep time: 10 minutes | **Cook time:** 15 minutes | **Yield:** 4 servings

Ingredients

- 2 eggs
- 1 teaspoon cream cheese
- 1 oz Parmesan, grated
- ¼ teaspoon red pepper
- 1 oz bacon, chopped
- 1 cup of water

Method

1. Pour water in the instant pot.

2. Add eggs and cook them for 5 minutes on manual mode (high pressure).

3. Then make a quick pressure release. Cool and peel the eggs.

4. After this, clean the instant pot bowl and put the bacon inside.

5. Cook it on saute mode for 10 minutes. Stir it from time to time to avoid burning.

6. Cut the eggs into halves.

7. Put the egg yolks in the bowl and smash them with the help of the fork.

8. Add red pepper, cooked bacon, and cream cheese. Mix up the mixture.

9. Then fill the egg whites with the bacon mixture.

Nutritional info per serve: calories 98, fat 7, fiber 0.1, carbs 1.1, protein 7.8

Rosemary Chicken Wings

Prep time: 10 minutes | **Cook time:** 16 minutes | **Yield:** 4 servings

Ingredients

- 4 chicken wings, boneless
- 1 tablespoon olive oil
- 1 teaspoon dried

- rosemary
- ½ teaspoon garlic powder
- ¼ teaspoon salt

Method

1. In the mixing bowl, mix up olive oil, dried rosemary, garlic powder, and salt.

2. Then rub the chicken wings with the rosemary mixture and leave for 10 minutes to marinate.

3. After this, put the chicken wings in the instant pot, add the remaining rosemary marinade and cook them on saute mode for 8 minutes from each side.

Nutritional info per serve: calories 222, fat 11.1, fiber 0.2, carbs 1.8, protein 27.5

Classic Meatballs

Prep time: 20 minutes | **Cook time:** 15 minutes | **Yield:** 6 servings

Ingredients

- 7 oz ground beef
- 7 oz ground pork
- 1 teaspoon minced garlic
- 3 tablespoons water
- 1 teaspoon chili

- flakes
- 1 teaspoon dried parsley
- 1 tablespoon coconut oil
- ¼ cup beef broth

Method

1. In the mixing bowl, mix up ground beef, ground pork, minced garlic, water, chili flakes, and dried parsley.

2. Make the medium size meatballs from the mixture.

3. After this, heat up coconut oil in the instant pot on saute mode.

4. Put the meatballs in the hot coconut oil in one layer and cook them for 2 minutes from each side.

5. Then add beef broth and close the lid.

6. Cook the meatballs for 10 minutes on manual mode (high pressure).

7. Then make a quick pressure release and transfer the meatballs on the plate.

Nutritional info per serve: calories 131, fat 5.6, fiber 0, carbs 0.2, protein 18.9

Spinach Dip

Prep time: 10 minutes | **Cook time:** 6 hours | **Yield:** 4 servings

Ingredients

- 2 cups spinach, chopped
- 1 cup Mozzarella, shredded
- 2 artichoke hearts, chopped

- 1 teaspoon ground ginger
- 1 teaspoon butter
- ½ teaspoon white pepper
- ½ cup heavy cream

Method

1. Put the spinach, artichoke hearts, and butter in the instant pot bowl.

2. Add Mozzarella, ground ginger, white pepper, and heavy cream. Stir the mixture gently.

3. Cook it in manual mode (Low pressure) for 6 hours. Then stir well and transfer in the serving bowl.

Nutritional info per serve: calories 124, fat 8, fiber 4.8, carbs 10.2, protein 5.5

Cheese Stuffed Shishito Peppers

Prep time: 20 minutes | **Cook time:** 7 minutes | **Yield:** 4 servings

Ingredients

- 8 oz shishito peppers
- 1 cup Cheddar cheese, shredded
- 4 tablespoons cream cheese
- 1 tablespoon fresh parsley, chopped

- ¼ teaspoon minced garlic
- 1 tablespoon butter, melted
- 1 cup water, for cooking

Method

1. Cut the ends of the peppers and remove the seeds.

2. After this, in the mixing bowl mix up shredded cheese, cream cheese, parsley, and minced garlic.

3. Then fill the peppers with cheese mixture and put in the baking mold.

4. Sprinkle the peppers with melted butter.

5. After this, pour water and insert the steamer rack.

6. Place the mold with peppers on the rack. Close and seal the lid.

7. Cook the meal on manual (high pressure) for 7 minutes. Allow the natural pressure release for 5 minutes.

Nutritional info per serve: calories 194, fat 15.7, fiber 2.6, carbs 4.5, protein 9.1

Sausage Balls

Prep time: 10 minutes | **Cook time:** 16 minutes | **Yield:** 10 servings

Ingredients

- 15 oz ground pork sausage
- 1 teaspoon dried oregano
- 4 oz Mozzarella, shredded
- 1 cup coconut flour
- 1 garlic clove, grated
- 1 teaspoon coconut oil, melted

Method

1. In the bowl mix up ground pork sausages, dried oregano, shredded Mozzarella, coconut flour, and garlic clove.
2. When the mixture is homogenous, make the balls.
3. After this, pour coconut oil in the instant pot.
4. Arrange the balls in the instant pot and cook them on saute mode for 8 minutes from each side.

Nutritional info per serve: calories 310, fat 23.2, fiber 4.9, carbs 10.1, protein 16.8

BLT Dip

Prep time: 10 minutes | **Cook time:** 20 minutes | **Yield:** 3 servings

Ingredients

- 2 teaspoons cream cheese
- 3 oz bacon, chopped
- 2 tablespoons sour cream
- 2 oz Cheddar cheese, shredded
- ¼ teaspoon minced garlic
- 1 teaspoon smoked paprika
- 1 tomato, chopped
- ¼ cup lettuce, chopped

Method

1. Preheat the instant pot on saute mode.
2. Put the chopped bacon in the instant pot and cook it for 5 minutes. Stir it from time to time.
3. Then add cream cheese, sour cream, Cheddar cheese, garlic, smoked paprika, and tomato.
4. Close the lid and cook the dip on saute mode for 15 minutes.
5. Then stir it well and mix up with lettuce.

Nutritional info per serve: calories 261, fat 20.7, fiber 0.5, carbs 2.5, protein 15.9

Taco Bites

Prep time: 10 minutes | **Cook time:** 15 minutes | **Yield:** 6 servings

Ingredients

- 10 oz ground beef
- 3 eggs, beaten
- 1/3 cup Mozzarella, shredded
- 1 teaspoon taco seasoning
- 1 teaspoon sesame oil

Method

1. In the mixing bowl mix up ground beef, eggs, Mozzarella, and taco seasoning.
2. Then make the small meat bites from the mixture.
3. Heat up sesame oil in the instant pot.
4. Put the meat bites in the hot oil and cook them for 5 minutes from each side on Saute mode.

Nutritional info per serve: calories 132, fat 6.2, fiber 0, carbs 0.6, protein 17.5

Scallion Dip

Prep time: 10 minutes | **Cook time:** 11 minutes | **Yield:** 4 servings

Ingredients

- 5 oz scallions, diced
- 4 tablespoons cream cheese
- 1 tablespoon fresh parsley, chopped
- 1 teaspoon garlic
- powder
- 2 tablespoons coconut cream
- ½ teaspoon salt
- 1 teaspoon coconut oil

Method

1. Heat up the instant pot on saute mode.
2. Then add coconut oil and melt it.
3. Add diced scallions and saute it for 6-7 minutes or until it is light brown.
4. Add cream cheese, parsley, garlic powder, salt, and coconut cream.
5. Close the instant pot lid and cook the scallions dip for 5 minutes on Manual mode (high pressure).
6. Make a quick pressure release. Blend the dip will it is smooth if desired.

Nutritional info per serve: calories 76, fat 6.5, fiber 1.2, carbs 3.9, protein 1.7

Sausage Dip

Prep time: 10 minutes | **Cook time:** 25 minutes | **Yield:** 7 servings

Ingredients

- 12 oz Italian sausages
- 1 chili pepper, chopped
- 5 oz Cheddar cheese, shredded
- 1 teaspoon coconut oil
- 1 teaspoon tomato paste
- ¼ cup heavy cream

Method

1. Heat up coconut oil in the instant pot.
2. Then add Italian sausages and cook them on Saute mode for 10 minutes. Mix up the sausages every 3 minutes.
3. Then add chili pepper, shredded Cheddar cheese, tomato paste, and heavy cream.
4. Close the lid and cook the dip on manual mode (high pressure) for 10 minutes. Make a quick pressure release.

Nutritional info per serve: calories 271, fat 24.2, fiber 0.1, carbs 0.9, protein 12.1

Chicken Celery Sticks

Prep time: 15 minutes | **Cook time:** 15 minutes | **Yield:** 4 servings

Ingredients

- 14 oz chicken breast, skinless, boneless
- 1 cup of water
- 1 teaspoon salt
- ½ teaspoon onion powder
- 4 celery stalks
- 1 teaspoon Keto mayo

Method

1. Put the chicken breast in the instant pot.
2. Add water, salt, and onion powder.
3. Cook the chicken on manual mode (high pressure) for 15 minutes. Allow the natural pressure release for 6 minutes.
4. Remove the cooked chicken from the instant pot and shred it.
5. Add Keto mayo and stir well.
6. Fill the celery stalks with shredded chicken.

Nutritional info per serve: calories 118, fat 2.6, fiber 0.3, carbs 0.9, protein 21.2

Stuffed Mushrooms

Prep time: 15 minutes | **Cook time:** 8 minutes | **Yield:** 4 servings

Ingredients

- 1 cup cremini mushroom caps
- 1 tablespoon scallions, chopped
- 1 tablespoon chives, chopped
- 1 teaspoon cream cheese
- 1 teaspoon sour cream
- 1 oz Monterey Jack cheese, shredded
- 1 teaspoon butter, softened
- ½ teaspoon smoked paprika
- 1 cup water, for cooking

Method

1. Trim the mushroom caps if needed and wash them well.
2. After this, in the mixing bowl, mix up scallions, chives, cream cheese, sour cream, butter, and smoked paprika.
3. Then fill the mushroom caps with the cream cheese mixture and top with shredded Monterey Jack cheese.
4. Pour water and insert the trivet in the instant pot.
5. Arrange the stuffed mushrooms caps on the trivet and close the lid.
6. Cook the meal on Manual (high pressure) for 8 minutes.
7. Then make a quick pressure release.

Nutritional info per serve: calories 45, fat 3.7, fiber 0.3, carbs 1, protein 2.5

Red Cauliflower Rice

Prep time: 10 minutes | **Cook time:** 3 minutes | **Yield:** 4 servings

Ingredients

- 1 cup cauliflower, shredded
- 1 teaspoon tomato paste
- ½ cup coconut cream
- ½ teaspoon salt
- ¼ cup chicken broth
- 1 teaspoon dried cilantro

Method

1. Put all ingredients in the instant pot and stir until you get the red color of the cauliflower.
2. Close and seal the lid.
3. Cook the meal on manual (high pressure) for 3 minutes. Make a quick pressure release.

Nutritional info per serve: calories 79, fat 7.3, fiber 1.3, carbs 3.3, protein 1.6

Coconut Shrimps

Prep time: 10 minutes | **Cook time:** 6 minutes | **Yield:** 2 servings

Ingredients

- 4 Royal tiger shrimps
- 3 tablespoons coconut shred
- 2 eggs, beaten
- ½ teaspoon Cajun seasonings
- 1 teaspoon olive oil

Method

1. Heat up olive oil in the instant pot on saute mode.
2. Meanwhile, mix up Cajun seasonings and coconut shred.
3. Dip the shrimps in the eggs and coat in the coconut shred mixture.
4. After this, place the shrimps in the hot olive oil and cook them on saute mode for 3 minutes from each side.

Nutritional info per serve: calories 292, fat 53.7, fiber 1, carbs 2.3, protein 40.1

Eggplant Bites

Prep time: 15 minutes | **Cook time:** 20 minutes | **Yield:** 4 servings

Ingredients

- 1 teaspoon minced garlic
- 1 tablespoon apple cider vinegar
- 1 tablespoon sesame
- oil
- 1 teaspoon salt
- 2 large eggplants, trimmed
- 1 teaspoon dried sage

Method

1. Slice the eggplants and rub them with salt.
2. After this, in the shallow bowl mix up minced garlic, apple cider vinegar, sesame oil, and dried sage.
3. Then rub every eggplant slice with a minced garlic mixture.
4. Heat up the instant pot on saute mode.
5. Then place the eggplant slices in the instant pot in one layer. Cook the vegetables for 2 minutes from each side or until the eggplants are tender.

Nutritional info per serve: calories 101, fat 3.9, fiber 9.8, carbs 16.5, protein 2.8

Bacon Peppers

Prep time: 15 minutes | **Cook time:** 6 minutes | **Yield:** 2 servings

Ingredients

- 2 jalapenos
- 1 oz bacon, chopped, fried
- 1 teaspoon green onions, chopped
- 1 tablespoon coconut cream
- 2 oz Cheddar cheese, shredded

Method

1. Trim the jalapenos and remove the seeds.
2. In the mixing bowl, mix up chopped bacon, green onions, coconut cream, and shredded cheese.
3. Fill the jalapenos with the bacon mixture.
4. Heat up the instant pot on saute mode for 5 minutes.
5. Put the jalapenos in the instant pot and cook them for 3 minutes from each side.

Nutritional info per serve: calories 213, fat 17.2, fiber 0.6, carbs 1.9, protein 12.7

Fat Bombs

Prep time: 10 minutes | **Cook time:** 10 minutes | **Yield:** 3 servings

Ingredients

- 3 eggs
- 3 bacon slices
- ½ teaspoon cayenne pepper
- 2 tablespoons cream cheese
- ½ teaspoon salt

Method

1. Put the bacon in the instant pot and cook it on saute mode for 3 minutes from each side.
2. Then chop the bacon and put it in the bowl.
3. Crack the eggs in the instant pot and whisk gently.
4. Cook the eggs for 5 minutes on manual mode (high pressure). Make a quick pressure release.
5. Then transfer the cooked eggs in the bowl with bacon and shred.
6. Add cayenne pepper, cream cheese, and salt. Stir well.
7. Make the medium size bombs.

Nutritional info per serve: calories 190, fat 14.7, fiber 0.1, carbs 1, protein 13.1

Reuben Pickles

Prep time: 20 minutes | **Cook time:** 2 hours | **Yield:** 6 servings

Ingredients

- 1-pound corned beef brisket
- 2 cups of water
- 1 cup pickled cucumbers
- 2 oz provolone cheese, sliced

Method

1. Put corned beef brisket and water in the instant pot.

2. Cook the meat on manual mode (high pressure) for 2 hours. Allow the natural pressure release for 10 minutes.

3. Then remove the meat from water and slice it.

4. Make the Reuben pickles: pin the meat piece, pickled cucumber, and provolone cheese together to get the small bites.

   Nutritional info per serve: calories 164, fat 12, fiber 0.1, carbs 0.8, protein 12.7

Parmesan Balls with Greens

Prep time: 10 minutes | **Cook time:** 20 minutes | **Yield:** 4 servings

Ingredients

- 3 oz Parmesan, grated
- 1 cup ground chicken
- 1 tablespoon chives, chopped
- 1 teaspoon cayenne pepper
- ¼ cup chicken broth
- 1 teaspoon coconut oil, softened

Method

1. Heat up coconut oil in the instant pot on saute mode.

2. Add ground chicken, cayenne pepper, chives, and chicken broth.

3. Close the lid and cook the chicken on manual mode (high pressure) for 15 minutes.

4. Then make a quick pressure release and open the lid.

5. Add Parmesan and stir the chicken mixture well.

6. Make the balls from the cooked mixture and cool them for 10 minutes before serving.

   Nutritional info per serve: calories 149, fat 8.5, fiber 0.1, carbs 1.1, protein 17.3

Roasted Tomatillos

Prep time: 10 minutes | **Cook time:** 10 minutes | **Yield:** 4 servings

Ingredients

- 1 tablespoon Italian seasonings
- 4 tomatillos, sliced
- 4 teaspoons olive oil
- 4 tablespoons water

Method

1. Sprinkle the tomatillos with Italian seasoning.

2. Then pour the olive oil in the instant pot and heat it up on saute mode for 1 minute.

3. Put the tomatillos in the instant pot in one layer and cook them for 2 minutes from each side.

4. Then add water and close the lid.

5. Saute the vegetables for 3 minutes more.

   Nutritional info per serve: calories 51, fat 5, fiber 0.7, carbs 2, protein 0.3

Sesame Bok Choy

Prep time: 5 minutes | **Cook time:** 7 minutes | **Yield:** 2 servings

Ingredients

- 2 cups bok choy, sliced
- 1 teaspoon sesame seeds
- 1 tablespoon apple cider vinegar
- 1 teaspoon sesame oil
- ¾ teaspoon salt
- 1 cup water, for cooking

Method

1. Pour water and insert the steamer rack in the instant pot.

2. Put the bok choy in the steamer rack and close the lid.

3. Cook the vegetables on the "Steam" mode for 3 minutes.

4. Make a quick pressure release and transfer the bok choy on the plate.

5. Sprinkle the meal with salt, sesame oil, apple cider vinegar, and sesame seeds.

6. Shake the bok choy gently.

7. Serve the bok choy warm!

   Nutritional info per serve: calories 35, fat 2.9, fiber 0.7, carbs 1.8, protein 1.3

Steamed Kohlrabi

Prep time: 5 minutes | **Cook time:** 8 minutes | **Yield:** 5 servings

Ingredients

- 14 oz kohlrabi, chopped
- ½ garlic clove, diced
- 1 tablespoon avocado oil
- ½ teaspoon salt
- ½ cup chicken broth

Method

1. Pour avocado oil in the instant pot and add diced garlic.

2. Saute the ingredients for 3 minutes.

3. Add chopped kohlrabi and cook the greens for 2 minutes more.

4. After this, sprinkle them with salt and add chicken broth.

5. Close and seal the lid and cook the meal on the "steam" mode for 3 minutes.

6. Make a quick pressure release.

   Nutritional info per serve: calories 29, fat 0.6, fiber 3, carbs 5.3, protein 1.9

Chicken&Chinese Cabbage Salad

Prep time: 15 minutes | **Cook time:** 10 minutes | **Yield:** 4 servings

Ingredients

- 12 oz chicken fillet, chopped
- 1 teaspoon Cajun seasonings
- 1 tablespoon coconut oil
- 1 cup Chinese cabbage, chopped
- 1 tablespoon avocado oil
- 1 teaspoon sesame seeds

Method

1. Sprinkle the chopped chicken with Cajun seasonings and put in the instant pot.

2. Add coconut oil and cook the chicken on saute mode for 10 minutes. Stir it from time to time with the help of a spatula.

3. When the chicken is cooked, transfer it in the salad bowl.

4. Add Chinese cabbage, avocado oil, and sesame seeds.

5. Mix up the salad.

   Nutritional info per serve: calories 202, fat 10.6, fiber 0.4, carbs 0.8, protein 25

Cauliflower Fritters

Prep time: 10 minutes | **Cook time:** 10 minutes | **Yield:** 4 servings

Ingredients

- 1 cup cauliflower, boiled
- 2 oz Cheddar cheese, shredded
- 2 tablespoons almond flour
- ½ teaspoon garlic powder
- 2 eggs, beaten
- 1 tablespoon avocado oil

Method

1. Mash the cauliflower and mix it up with Cheddar cheese, almond flour, garlic powder, and eggs.

2. Heat up the avocado oil on saute mode for 1 minute.

3. Meanwhile, make the fritters from the cauliflower mixture.

4. Put them in the hot oil and cook for 3 minutes from each side.

   Nutritional info per serve: calories 122, fat 9, fiber 1.2, carbs 2.9, protein 7.7

Zucchini Cheese Tots

Prep time: 15 minutes | **Cook time:** 10 minutes | **Yield:** 6 servings

Ingredients

- 4 oz Parmesan, grated
- 4 oz Cheddar cheese, grated
- 1 zucchini, grated
- 1 egg, beaten
- 1 teaspoon dried oregano
- 1 tablespoon coconut oil

Method

1. In the mixing bowl, mix up Parmesan, Cheddar cheese, zucchini, egg, and dried oregano.

2. Make the small tots with the help of the fingertips.

3. Then melt the coconut oil in the instant pot on saute mode.

4. Put the prepared zucchini tots in the hot coconut oil and cook them for 3 minutes from each side or until they are light brown.

5. Cool the zucchini tots for 5 minutes.

   Nutritional info per serve: calories 173, fat 13.4, fiber 0.5, carbs 2.2, protein 12.1

Steamed Spinach with Garlic

Prep time: 5 minutes | **Cook time:** 4 minutes | **Yield:** 4 servings

Ingredients

- 2 cups spinach, chopped
- 1 cup organic almond milk
- 1 teaspoon minced
- garlic
- 1 tablespoon butter
- ½ teaspoon salt
- 2 oz Monterey Jack cheese, shredded

Method

1. Put all ingredients in the instant pot and stir gently.
2. Close and seal the lid.
3. Cook the meal on manual mode (high pressure) for 4 minutes. Make a quick pressure release.
4. After this, open the lid and stir the spinach well.

Nutritional info per serve: calories 98, fat 7.9, fiber 0.3, carbs 2.9, protein 4.2

Feta Psiti

Prep time: 10 minutes | **Cook time:** 6 minutes | **Yield:** 6 servings

Ingredients

- 12 oz Feta cheese
- ½ tomato, sliced
- 1 oz bell pepper, sliced
- 1 teaspoon ground paprika
- 1 tablespoon olive oil
- 1 cup water, for cooking

Method

1. Sprinkle the cheese with olive oil and ground paprika and place it on the foil.
2. Then top Feta cheese with sliced tomato and bell pepper. Wrap it in the foil well.
3. After this, pour water and insert the steamer rack in the instant pot.
4. Put the wrapped cheese on the rack. Close and seal the lid.
5. Cook the cheese on manual mode (high pressure) for 6 minutes. Then make a quick pressure release.
6. Discard the foil and transfer the cheese on the serving plates.

Nutritional info per serve: calories 178, fat 14.5, fiber 0.5, carbs 4.2, protein 8.4

Lemon Mushrooms

Prep time: 10 minutes | **Cook time:** 4 minutes | **Yield:** 2 servings

Ingredients

- 1 cup cremini mushrooms, sliced
- 1 teaspoon lemon zest, grated
- 1 tablespoon lemon juice
- ½ teaspoon salt
- ½ teaspoon dried thyme
- ½ cup of water
- 1 teaspoon almond butter

Method

1. Put all ingredients in the instant pot and stir them with the help of the spatula.
2. Then close and seal the instant pot lid.
3. Cook the mushrooms on manual mode (high pressure) for 4 minutes.
4. When the time of cooking is finished, allow the natural pressure release for 5 minutes.

Nutritional info per serve: calories 62, fat 4.6, fiber 1.2, carbs 3.5, protein 2.7

Sesame Broccoli Sprouts

Prep time: 5 minutes | **Cook time:** 1 minute | **Yield:** 4 servings

Ingredients

- 1-pound broccoli sprouts
- 1 cup of water
- 1 teaspoon coconut aminos
- ½ teaspoon chili
- pepper, chopped
- ½ teaspoon salt
- 1 teaspoon minced garlic
- 1 teaspoon sesame oil

Method

1. Pour water in the instant pot. Close the lid.
2. Bring the water to boil on saute mode (appx. 10 minutes).
3. Then open the lid and add broccoli sprouts. Leave the sprouts in the hot water for 1 minute.
4. Then transfer the sprouts in the bowl.
5. In the separated bowl, mix up coconut aminos, chili pepper, salt, minced garlic, and sesame oil.
6. Pour mixture over the broccoli sprouts. Shake the greens.

Nutritional info per serve: calories 53, fat 1.1, fiber 4, carbs 4.6, protein 4.1

Faux-Tatoes

Prep time: 5 minutes | **Cook time:** 18 minutes | **Yield:** 4 servings

Ingredients

- 1 daikon radish, sliced
- 3 oz scallions, diced
- 1 tablespoon coconut oil
- 1 teaspoon salt

Method

1. Mix up daikon radish and scallions in the bowl and sprinkle with salt.
2. Then toss the coconut oil in the instant pot and melt it on saute mode.
3. Add daikon radish mixture and close the lid.
4. Saute the vegetables for 5 minutes and turn into another side.
5. Cook the vegetables for 10 minutes more. Stir them from time to time.

Nutritional info per serve: calories 39, fat 3.4, fiber 0.8, carbs 2.1, protein 0.6

Broccoli Skewers

Prep time: 15 minutes | **Cook time:** 1 minute | **Yield:** 2 servings

Ingredients

- 1 cup broccoli florets
- ½ teaspoon curry paste
- 2 tablespoons coconut cream
- 1 cup water, for cooking

Method

1. In the shallow bowl mix up curry paste and coconut cream.
2. Then sprinkle the broccoli florets with curry paste mixture and string on the skewers.
3. Pour water and insert the steamer rack in the instant pot.
4. Place the broccoli skewers on the rack. Close and seal the lid.
5. Cook the meal on manual mode (high pressure) for 1 minute.
6. Make a quick pressure release.

Nutritional info per serve: calories 58, fat 4.5, fiber 1.5, carbs 4.2, protein 1.7

Garlic Shirataki Noodles

Prep time: 10 minutes | **Cook time:** 3 minutes | **Yield:** 4 servings

Ingredients

- 7 oz shirataki noodles
- 1 garlic clove, minced
- 1 tablespoon olive oil
- 1 teaspoon fresh cilantro, chopped
- 1 cup hot water

Method

1. Put shirataki noodles in the hot water and leave them for 3 minutes.
2. Meanwhile, pour olive oil in the instant pot.
3. Add minced garlic and saute it for 2 minutes.
4. Stir well.
5. After this, remove the noodles from water and transfer in the instant pot.
6. Add chopped cilantro and stir well. Cook the meal for 1 minute more.

Nutritional info per serve: calories 42, fat 3.5, fiber 5.3, carbs 0.3, protein 0.4

Steamed Fennel Bulb

Prep time: 10 minutes | **Cook time:** 7 minutes | **Yield:** 2 servings

Ingredients

- 8 oz fennel bulb, chopped
- 1 teaspoon olive oil
- 1 teaspoon
- ¼ teaspoon cayenne pepper
- ¼ teaspoon
- 1 cup water, for cooking

Method

1. Pour water and insert the steamer rack in the instant pot.
2. Place the chopped fennel in the steamer rack. Close and seal the lid.
3. Cook the vegetables on steam mode for 7 minutes. Make a quick pressure release.
4. After this, transfer the fennel in the bog bowl and sprinkle with olive oil, coconut aminos, cayenne pepper, and Splenda.
5. Mix up the vegetables well.

Nutritional info per serve: calories 61, fat 2.6, fiber 3.6, carbs 9.4, protein 1.4

Shrimp Sandwich

Prep time: 5 minutes | **Cook time:** 5 minutes | **Yield:** 2 servings

Ingredients

- 4 lettuce leaves
- 4 king shrimps, peeled
- 1 teaspoon lemon juice
- ½ teaspoon white pepper
- 2 tablespoons butter
- ½ teaspoon salt

Method

1. Sprinkle the shrimps with white pepper and salt and put in the instant pot.
2. Add butter and cook the seafood for 3 minutes on saute mode.
3. Then flip the shrimps on another side and cook them for 2 minutes more.
4. Sprinkle the cooked shrimps with lemon juice and transfer on lettuce leaves (2 shrimps per one lettuce leaf).
5. Cover them with the remaining lettuce.

Nutritional info per serve: calories 165, fat 12.6, fiber 0.2, carbs 0.7, protein 12.3

Cheese Chips

Prep time: 10 minutes | **Cook time:** 5 minutes | **Yield:** 4 servings

Ingredients

- 1 cup cheddar cheese, shredded
- 1 tablespoon almond flour

Method

1. Mix up cheddar cheese and almond flour.
2. Then preheat the instant pot on saute mode.
3. Line the instant pot bowl with baking paper.
4. After this, make the small rounds from the cheese in the instant pot (on the baking paper) and close the lid.
5. Cook them for 5 minutes on saute mode or until the cheese is melted.
6. Then switch off the instant pot and remove the baking paper with cheese rounds from it.
7. Cool the chips well and remove them from the baking paper.

Nutritional info per serve: calories 154, fat 12.9, fiber 0.8, carbs 1.9, protein 8.5

Cheese Bombs

Prep time: 15 minutes | **Cook time:** 15 minutes | **Yield:** 4 servings

Ingredients

- ¼ cup Mozzarella, shredded
- 1 egg, beaten
- ½ cup almond flour
- 1 teaspoon butter, softened
- 1 cup water, for cooking

Method

1. Grease the baking pan with butter.
2. After this, in the mixing bowl mix up Mozzarella, egg, and almond flour.
3. Make the small balls from the mixture and put them in the prepared baking pan.
4. After this, pour water in the instant pot and insert the steamer rack.
5. Place the baking pan with cheese bombs in the instant pot. Close and seal the lid.
6. Cook the meal on manual mode (high pressure) for 15 minutes. Make a quick pressure release.

Nutritional info per serve: calories 49, fat 4.1, fiber 0.4, carbs 0.9, protein 2.6

Zucchini Fries

Prep time: 15 minutes | **Cook time:** 5 minutes | **Yield:** 4 servings

Ingredients

- 1 zucchini
- 1 oz Parmesan, grated
- 1 tablespoon almond flour
- ½ teaspoon Italian seasonings
- 1 tablespoon coconut oil

Method

1. Trim the zucchini and cut it into the French fries.
2. Then sprinkle them with grated parmesan, almond flour, and Italian seasonings.
3. Put coconut oil in the instant pot and melt it on saute mode.
4. Put the zucchini in the hot oil in one layer and cook for 2 minutes from each side or until they are golden brown.
5. Dry the zucchini fries with paper towels.

Nutritional info per serve: calories 102, fat 8.7, fiber 1.3, carbs 3.5, protein 4.4

Rangoon Crab Dip

Prep time: 10 minutes | **Cook time:** 3 hours | **Yield:** 3 servings

Ingredients

- ½ cup Monterey jack cheese, shredded
- 6 oz crab meat, chopped
- ½ cup of coconut milk
- 1 tablespoon scallions, chopped
- ½ teaspoon garlic powder
- 1 teaspoon butter, softened

Method

1. Put the crab meat, coconut milk, scallions, and garlic powder in the instant pot.
2. Stir the mixture and add butter.
3. Then top it with cheese and close the lid.
4. Cook the dip on Low for 3 hours.

   Nutritional info per serve: calories 226, fat 17.5, fiber 1, carbs 3.9, protein 12.8

Zucchini and Cheese Scones

Prep time: 15 minutes | **Cook time:** 20 minutes | **Yield:** 4 servings

Ingredients

- ½ cup zucchini, grated
- ¼ cup Cheddar cheese, shredded
- 1 egg, beaten
- ¼ cup coconut flour
- ½ teaspoon ground black pepper
- 1 cup water, for cooking

Method

1. Make the dough: mix up zucchini, cheese, egg, coconut flour, and ground black pepper.
2. Then transfer the mixture in the non-stick baking pan and flatten well.
3. Pour water and insert the rack in the instant pot.
4. Put the pan with zucchini mixture on the rack. Close and seal the lid.
5. Cook the meal on manual mode (high pressure) for 20 minutes.
6. Make a quick pressure release.
7. Cool the cooked zucchini meal well and cut into the scones.

   Nutritional info per serve: calories 71, fat 3.7, fiber 3.5, carbs 6.2, protein 3.9

Steamed Savoy Cabbage

Prep time: 5 minutes | **Cook time:** 7 minutes | **Yield:** 4 servings

Ingredients

- 1-pound savoy cabbage, chopped
- 1/3 cup butter
- 1 teaspoon salt
- ½ teaspoon white pepper
- 1 cup chicken broth

Method

1. Put all ingredients in the instant pot and stir them well.
2. After this, close and seal the lid.
3. Cook the savoy cabbage on manual mode (high pressure) for 7 minutes.
4. Then make a quick pressure release and open the lid.
5. Stir the meal well before serving.

   Nutritional info per serve: calories 174, fat 15.8, fiber 2.9, carbs 7, protein 2.9

Flax Meal Bread

Prep time: 20 minutes | **Cook time:** 20 minutes | **Yield:** 4 servings

Ingredients

- 1 egg, beaten
- 2 tablespoons cream cheese
- ½ cup coconut flour
- 3 tablespoons flax meal
- ¼ teaspoon baking powder
- 1 teaspoon lemon juice
- 1 teaspoon butter
- 1 cup water, for cooking

Method

1. Mix up egg, cream cheese, coconut flour, flax meal, baking powder, lemon juice, and knead the dough.
2. Then grease the bread mold with butter and transfer the dough inside.
3. Flatten it in the shape of the bread.
4. Then pour water in the instant pot and insert the bread mold.
5. Close and seal the lid.
6. Cook the bread on manual mode (high pressure) for 20 minutes and then do the quick pressure release.
7. Cool the bread to the room temperature and slice it.

   Nutritional info per serve: calories 135, fat 8.2, fiber 7.5, carbs 10.9, protein 5.9

Zucchini Ravioli

Prep time: 15 minutes | **Cook time:** 20 minutes | **Yield:** 2 servings

Ingredients

- 1 zucchini, trimmed
- 1 tablespoon ricotta cheese
- 2 oz spinach, chopped
- 1 teaspoon olive oil
- 1 garlic clove, minced
- ¼ cup keto marinara sauce
- ¼ cup chicken broth

Method

1. Slice the zucchini into vertical slices with the help of the potato peeler.
2. Then heat up olive oil on saute mode for 1 minute.
3. Add spinach and garlic. Cook it for 3 minutes and transfer in the bowl.
4. Add ricotta cheese.
5. Make the cross from 4 zucchini slices and put the small amount of the ricotta cheese mixture inside. Wrap the zucchini into the balls and place them in the instant pot in one layer.
6. Add chicken broth and marinara sauce.
7. Close the lid and saute the meal for 15 minutes on saute mode.

   Nutritional info per serve: calories 87, fat 4.3, fiber 2.5, carbs 9.6, protein 4.2

Cheese and Mushrooms Cakes

Prep time: 15 minutes | **Cook time:** 10 minutes | **Yield:** 3 servings

Ingredients

- 7 oz white mushrooms, grinded
- 1 teaspoon butter
- 1/3 teaspoon salt
- 1 egg, beaten
- ¾ teaspoon chili pepper
- 3 oz Cheddar cheese, shredded

Method

1. Mix up all the ingredients together, except the butter.
2. Heat up butter on saute mode.
3. Then make the small cakes from the mushroom mixture and put them in the hot butter.
4. Cook the meal on saute mode for 4 minutes from each side.

   Nutritional info per serve: calories 161, fat 12.3, fiber 0.7, carbs 2.8, protein 11

Eggplant Parm

Prep time: 15 minutes | **Cook time:** 10 minutes | **Yield:** 2 servings

Ingredients

- 1 eggplant, sliced
- 1 teaspoon dried basil
- 1/3 cup keto marinara sauce
- ¼ cup Mozzarella, shredded
- 1 tablespoon butter
- ½ cup beef broth

Method

1. Grease the instant pot bowl with butter.
2. Then place the layer of the sliced eggplants in the instant pot and sprinkle it with shredded cheese and dried basil.
3. Repeat the step one more time.
4. Add beef broth and keto marinara sauce.
5. Close and seal the lid and cook the eggplant parm for 10 minutes.
6. Make a quick pressure release and cool the meal for 5 minutes before serving.

   Nutritional info per serve: calories 140, fat 7.7, fiber 8.4, carbs 15.5, protein 4.5

Cream Cheese Puree

Prep time: 8 minutes | **Cook time:** 5 minutes | **Yield:** 2 servings

Ingredients

- 1 cup of water
- ½ teaspoon salt
- 2 tablespoons cream
- cheese
- 10 oz cauliflower, chopped

Method

1. Place the chopped cauliflower in the instant pot.
2. Add salt and water.
3. Set the "Manual" mode (High pressure) on the instant pot.
4. Set the timer for 5 minutes.
5. When the time is over – use the quick pressure release method.
6. Transfer the cauliflower (without liquid) in the blender. Blend it until smooth.
7. After this, transfer the cauliflower mash in the bowl. Add cream cheese and stir the puree until homogenous.

   Nutritional info per serve: calories 70, fat 3.6, fiber 3.5, carbs 7.8, protein 3.6

Butter Zoodles

Prep time: 15 minutes | **Cook time:** 10 minutes | **Yield:** 2 servings

Ingredients

- 1 cup of water
- 1 large zucchini
- 2 tablespoons butter, softened

Method

1. Make the zoodles from zucchini with the help of the spiralizer.
2. Then pour water in the instant pot and bring it to boil on saute mode.
3. Then add zucchini zoodles and let them cook for 1 minute.
4. Remove the zoodles from water and add butter. Stir well.

Nutritional info per serve: calories 128, fat 11.8, fiber 1.8, carbs 5.4, protein 2.1

Garlic Asparagus

Prep time: 6 minutes | **Cook time:** 4 minutes | **Yield:** 2 servings

Ingredients

- 9 oz asparagus
- ½ teaspoon garlic powder
- 1 teaspoon butter
- ¾ teaspoon minced garlic
- 2 oz Parmesan, shredded
- 1 cup water, for cooking

Method

1. Grease the springform pan with butter.
2. Place the asparagus in the springform pan.
3. Sprinkle the vegetables with the garlic powder, and minced garlic.
4. Add water in the instant pot. Insert the springform with asparagus inside.
5. Close the lid and set the "Manual" mode (High pressure) for 4 minutes.
6. When the asparagus is cooked – make quick pressure release.
7. Transfer the asparagus on the serving plates immediately and sprinkle with the shredded cheese.

Nutritional info per serve: calories 137, fat 8.2, fiber 2.8, carbs 6.8, protein 12.1

Garlic Butter with Herbs

Prep time: 10 minutes | **Cook time:** 8 minutes | **Yield:** 4 servings

Ingredients

- 1/3 cup butter
- 1 teaspoon dried parsley
- 1 tablespoon dried dill
- ½ teaspoon minced garlic
- ¼ teaspoon dried thyme

Method

1. Preheat the instant pot on saute mode.
2. Then add butter and melt it.
3. Add dried parsley, dill, minced garlic, and thyme. Stir the butter mixture well.
4. Transfer it in the butter mold and refrigerate until it is solid.

Nutritional info per serve: calories 138, fat 15.4, fiber 0.2, carbs 0.6, protein 0.4

Brussel Sprouts Hash

Prep time: 6 minutes | **Cook time:** 9 minutes | **Yield:** 2 servings

Ingredients

- 1 cup Brussel sprouts, chopped
- 1 egg, beaten
- 2 oz Parmesan cheese, shredded
- 1 tablespoon butter, melted

Method

1. Combine together the chopped Brussel sprouts and beaten egg. Stir the mixture until homogenous.
2. Add shredded cheese and butter.
3. Stir the mixture with the help of a spatula.
4. After this, transfer the mixture in the non-sticky springform pan or cake mold.
5. Pour water in the instant pot.
6. Place the pan in the instant pot.
7. Lock the instant pot lid and seal it.
8. Set the "Manual" mode – High Pressure.
9. Cook hash brown for 4 minutes. Then make naturally pressure release for 5 minutes.

Nutritional info per serve: calories 192, fat 14.2, fiber 1.7, carbs 5.2, protein 13.4

Marjoram Cauliflower Florets

Prep time: 5 minutes | **Cook time:** 1 minute | **Yield:** 2 servings

Ingredients

- 1 teaspoon butter
- ½ teaspoon salt
- 1 teaspoon dried marjoram
- ½ cup beef broth
- 10 oz cauliflower

Method

1. Cut the cauliflower into the florets and sprinkle with the dried marjoram and salt.
2. Transfer the vegetables in the instant pot.
3. Add butter and beef broth.
4. Close the lid and set "Manual" mode (High pressure); cook the meal for 1 minute.
5. Then make quick pressure release and open the lid.
6. Add the butter in the cauliflower.

   Nutritional info per serve: calories 63, fat 2.4, fiber 3.7, carbs 7.9, protein 4.1

Broccoli Puree

Prep time: 10 minutes | **Cook time:** 6 minutes | **Yield:** 2 servings

Ingredients

- 7 oz broccoli, chopped
- ½ cup heavy cream

Method

1. Pour heavy cream in the instant pot.
2. Add broccoli and close the lid.
3. Cook the vegetables on manual mode (high pressure) for 6 minutes of +quick pressure release.
4. Transfer the broccoli and ¼ part of all liquid in the blender and blend the mixture until you get a smooth puree.

   Nutritional info per serve: calories 137, fat 11.4, fiber 2.6, carbs 7.4, protein 3.4

Sauteed Green Mix

Prep time: 5 minutes | **Cook time:** 10 minutes | **Yield:** 2 servings

Ingredients

- 2 cups spinach, chopped
- 1 cup kale, chopped
- ½ cup chicken stock
- 1 teaspoon cream cheese
- ½ teaspoon salt
- ½ cup broccoli raab, chopped

Method

1. Pour the chicken stock in the instant pot bowl.
2. Add cream cheese, salt, spinach, kale, and broccoli raab.
3. Cook the meal on the "Saute" mode for 5 minutes. Stir well.
4. Discard the greens from the chicken stock gravy and transfer on the plates.

   Nutritional info per serve: calories 37, fat 0.8, fiber 1.2, carbs 5.6, protein 2.7

Chili Zoodles

Prep time: 7 minutes | **Cook time:** 3 minutes | **Yield:** 2 servings

Ingredients

- 1 teaspoon chili flakes
- 2 zucchini
- ½ cup chicken stock
- 1 teaspoon coconut oil

Method

1. Make the noodles from the zucchini with the help of the spiralizer.
2. Sprinkle zucchini noodles with the salt and chili flakes.
3. Place the chicken stock and coconut oil in the instant pot bowl and preheat the liquid on the "Saute" mode.
4. Add the spiralized zucchini and cook on "Manual" mode - Zero –QPR.
5. The meal is cooked.

   Nutritional info per serve: calories 54, fat 2.8, fiber 2.2, carbs 6.8, protein 2.6

Ginger Cabbage

Prep time: 7 minutes | **Cook time:** 15 minutes | **Yield:** 2 servings

Ingredients

- ½ tablespoon ginger paste
- 10 oz white cabbage, shredded
- 1 teaspoon butter
- ½ cup heavy cream
- ½ teaspoon salt

Method

1. Place the cabbage in the big mixing bowl.
2. Sprinkle the cabbage with the ginger paste and salt.
3. Melt the butter on the "Saute" mode in the instant pot.
4. Then add all the shredded cabbage and heavy cream.
5. Set the "steam" mode and cook the cabbage for 10 minutes.
6. Transfer the cooked meal on the serving plates and enjoy!

    Nutritional info per serve: calories 160, fat 13.2, fiber 3.7, carbs 10, protein 2.6

Italian Style Kale

Prep time: 5 minutes | **Cook time:** 3 minutes | **Yield:** 3 servings

Ingredients

- 10 oz kale, Italian dark-leaf
- 1 tablespoon Italian
- seasonings
- 1 cup water, for cooking

Method

1. Chop the kale roughly and put it in the steamer pan. Sprinkle the greens with seasonings and stir well.
2. Then pour water and insert the steamer rack in the instant pot.
3. Put the pan with kale in the instant pot.
4. Cook the meal on the "Steam" mode for 3 minutes.

    Nutritional info per serve: calories 61, fat 1.4, fiber 1.4, carbs 10.4, protein 2.8

Parsley Fennel

Prep time: 10 minutes | **Cook time:** 5 minutes | **Yield:** 2 servings

Ingredients

- 1 fennel bulb, sliced
- ¾ cup fresh parsley, chopped
- 1 cup of water
- 1 teaspoon apple cider vinegar
- 1 tablespoon coconut aminos
- 1 tablespoon olive oil

Method

1. Pour water and insert the steamer rack in the instant pot.
2. Put the sliced fennel inside and cook it on Steam mode for 5 minutes.
3. Then transfer the fennel in the big bowl and sprinkle with apple cider vinegar, parsley, and olive oil.
4. Shake the fenne gently.

    Nutritional info per serve: calories 112, fat 7.4, fiber 4.4, carbs 11.5, protein 2.1

Lemon Flavored Broccoli

Prep time: 10 minutes | **Cook time:** 18 minutes | **Yield:** 2 servings

Ingredients

- 1 teaspoon salt
- 8 oz broccoli
- ¾ cup cream cheese
- ¼ cup of water
- 1 teaspoon grated lemon

Method

1. Cut the broccoli into the medium pieces and place them in the instant pot.
2. Add cream cheese and start to saute it for 3 minutes on the "Saute" mode.
3. Then add salt and grated lemon.
4. Stir gently and close the lead. Cook the meal on "Saute mode" for 15 minutes.
5. Serve the broccoli with a small amount of gravy.

    Nutritional info per serve: calories 343, fat 30.7, fiber 3, carbs 10.1, protein 9.8

Celery Stalk Chicken Salad

Prep time: 10- minutes | **Cook time:** 15 minutes | **Yield:** 2 servings

Ingredients

- 7 oz celery stalks, chopped
- 4 oz chicken fillet
- 1 teaspoon ground
- black pepper
- ½ teaspoon salt
- 1 cup of water

Method

1. Put the chicken in the instant pot. Add water and ground black pepper.

2. Cook the chicken on manual mode (high pressure) for 15 minutes + QPR.

3. Then shred the chicken and mix it up with salt and chopped celery stalk.

   Nutritional info per serve: calories 144, fat 6.1, fiber 1.9, carbs 3.8, protein 17.6

Salmon Salad with Feta

Prep time: 10 minutes | **Cook time:** 4 minutes | **Yield:** 2 servings

Ingredients

- 2 oz Feta, crumbled
- 6 oz salmon
- 1 cup lettuce, chopped
- 1 teaspoon olive oil
- ½ teaspoon salt
- 1 cup water, for cooking

Method

1. Sprinkle the salmon with salt and wrap in foil.

2. Place the salmon on the trivet and transfer it in the instant pot bowl.

3. Add 1 cup of water in the instant pot bowl and close the lid.

4. Cook the salmon on "Manual" mode (High Pressure) for 4 minutes (QR).

5. Meanwhile, tear the lettuce and toss it in the salad bowl.

6. Sprinkle it with olive oil.

7. When the salmon is cooked, chop it roughly and add in the lettuce.

8. Add crumbled Feta and shake the salad.

   Nutritional info per serve: calories 211, fat 13.7, fiber 0.2, carbs 2, protein 20.7

Tender Purple Petals

Prep time: 10 minutes | **Cook time:** 5 minutes | **Yield:** 2 servings

Ingredients

- 7 oz purple cabbage
- ¼ teaspoon salt
- 1 teaspoon butter
- ½ cup chicken broth

Method

1. Cut the cabbage into the petals and sprinkle with salt.

2. Place the cabbage into the instant pot.

3. Add butter and chicken broth.

4. Close the lid and set the "Steam" mode 5 minutes. Then make quick pressure release.

   Nutritional info per serve: calories 51, fat 2.4, fiber 2.5, carbs 6, protein 2.5

Zucchini Cheese Rings

Prep time: 15 minutes | **Cook time:** 3 minutes | **Yield:** 2 servings

Ingredients

- 1 zucchini
- 1 cup cheddar cheese, shredded
- 2 teaspoon butter, softened
- 2 cup of water

Method

1. Cut the zucchini into rings and remove the center of every ring.

2. Then grease the baking pan with softened butter and place the zucchini inside in one layer.

3. Fill every vegetable ring with shredded cheese.

4. After this, pour water and insert the trivet in the instant pot.

5. Put the baking pan with zucchini rings on the trivet.

6. Close and seal the lid.

7. Cook the meal on manual mode (high pressure) for 3 minutes. Then make a quick pressure release.

8. Cool the zucchini rings for 5-7 minutes before serving.

   Nutritional info per serve: calories 277, fat 22.7, fiber 1.1, carbs 4, protein 15.3

Scrambled Eggs Salad

Prep time: 10 minutes | **Cook time:** 5 minutes | **Yield:** 2 servings

Ingredients

- 1 tomato, chopped
- 2 eggs
- 2 tablespoons coconut milk
- 1 teaspoon butter
- 1 bell pepper, chopped

Method

1. Heat up butte on saute mode.
2. Crack the eggs in the butter.
3. Add coconut milk and stir the egg mixture until smooth. Saute it for 2 minutes and then scramble again. Cook the eggs for 2 minutes more and transfer in the bowl.
4. Add tomato and bell pepper.
5. Mix up the salad.

Nutritional info per serve: calories 139, fat 10.1, fiber 1.5, carbs 6.9, protein 6.8

Turmeric Cauliflower Shred

Prep time: 5 minutes | **Cook time:** 5 minutes | **Yield:** 2 servings

Ingredients

- ½ cup chicken broth
- 8 oz cauliflower, shredded
- 1 teaspoon butter
- 1 teaspoon ground turmeric

Method

1. Put the butter in the instant pot and preheat it on the "Saute" mode.
2. Add shredded cauliflower and salt. Stir the mixture and cook for 1 minute more.
3. After this, add chicken broth and turmeric, mix up the ingredients and lock the instant pot.
4. Set the "Manual" mode (High pressure) and cook the side dish for 1 minute.
5. After this, make a quick pressure release (follow the directions of your instant pot).

Nutritional info per serve: calories 59, fat 2.5, fiber 3.1, carbs 7, protein 3.6

Butter Konjac Noodles

Prep time: 10 minutes | **Cook time:** 1 minute | **Yield:** 2 servings

Ingredients

- 7 oz Konjac Noodles
- 1 teaspoon butter, melted
- 1 cup of water

Method

1. Pour water in the instant pot and bring it to boil on Saute mode.
2. Add konjac noodles and leave them in the water for 1 minute.
3. Then rinse the noodles and carefully mix them up with butter.

Nutritional info per serve: calories 26, fat 11.9, fiber 3, carbs 3.5, protein 0

Cream Keto Beans

Prep time: 5 minutes | **Cook time:** 3 minutes | **Yield:** 4 servings

Ingredients

- 2 teaspoons butter
- 11 oz green beans
- 1 cup coconut cream

Method

1. Put all ingredients in the instant pot
2. Set the "Manual" mode (High pressure) and put time for 2 minutes.
3. When the time is over – make quick pressure release.

Nutritional info per serve: calories 179, fat 16.3, fiber 4, carbs 8.9, protein 2.8

Tender Celery Cubes

Prep time: 6 minutes | **Cook time:** 15 minutes | **Yield:** 2 servings

Ingredients

- 1 cup celery root, chopped
- 1 garlic clove, chopped
- ½ teaspoon ground coriander
- ½ teaspoon salt
- ¾ teaspoon ground cinnamon
- ½ cup of coconut milk
- 1 teaspoon butter

Method

1. Put all ingredients in the instant pot.
2. Close and seal the lid.
3. Cook the ragout on the "Saute" mode for 15 minutes to get the soft vegetable texture.

Nutritional info per serve: calories 192, fat 16.5, fiber 3.2, carbs 11.7, protein 2.7

Kale Saute with Flax Seeds

Prep time: 5 minutes | **Cook time:** 4 minutes | **Yield:** 2 servings

Ingredients

- 1 cup Kale, Italian dark-leaf, chopped
- 1 teaspoon butter
- 1 tablespoon flax seeds
- ¾ teaspoon ground nutmeg
- 1 teaspoon olive oil
- ¼ cup of water

Method

1. Toss butter in the instant pot bowl and melt it on the "Saute" mode.

2. Add the chopped kale. Sprinkle the kale leaves with the salt and ground nutmeg.

3. Add water Stir the kale well.

4. Cook it on the "Saute" mode for 4 minutes.

5. Then transfer the cooked kale on the serving plates and sprinkle with the olive oil and flax seeds.

   Nutritional info per serve: calories 76, fat 5.4, fiber 1.6, carbs 4.9, protein 1.7

Cremini Mushrooms Stew

Prep time: 8 minutes | **Cook time:** 25 minutes | **Yield:** 2 servings

Ingredients

- 2 teaspoons butter
- 1 cup cremini mushrooms, sliced
- ½ cup heavy cream
- ½ teaspoon white pepper
- ¼ teaspoon turmeric

Method

1. Melt the butter in the instant pot bowl on the "Saute" mode.

2. Add heavy cream, white pepper, turmeric, and stir well.

3. Preheat the liquid until it starts to boil.

4. Add sliced mushrooms and stir well.

5. After this, close the lid and cook the saute on the "Saute" mode for 20 minutes. Reduce the time of cooking if you want the solid texture of the mushrooms.

   Nutritional info per serve: calories 149, fat 15, fiber 0.4, carbs 2.8, protein 1.60

Aromatic Eggplant Mix

Prep time: 5 minutes | **Cook time:** 30 minutes | **Yield:** 2 servings

Ingredients

- 8 oz eggplant, chopped
- 3 oz asparagus, chopped
- 1 teaspoon salt
- 1 teaspoon ground cumin
- 1 cup chicken broth
- 1 bell pepper, chopped

Method

1. Put all vegetables in the instant pot.

2. Close the lid and cook the meal on saute mode for 30 minutes.

3. When the time is finished and the meal is cooked, stir it well with the help of the spoon.

   Nutritional info per serve: calories 186, fat 12.1, fiber 4.9, carbs 11.2, protein 10.8

Soups & Stews

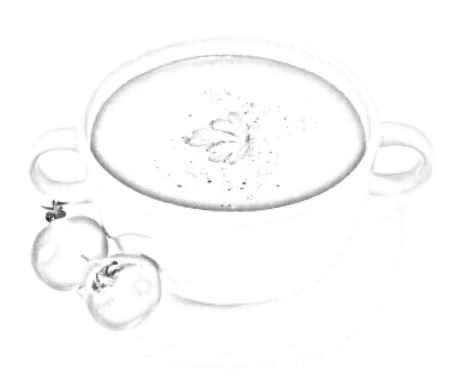

Broccoli Cheese Soup

Prep time: 10 minutes | **Cook time:** 5 minutes | **Yield:** 4 servings

Ingredients

- 2 cups broccoli florets
- 1 cup Cheddar cheese, shredded
- 2 garlic cloves, diced
- 1 tablespoon olive oil
- 1 cup heavy cream
- 2 cups chicken broth
- ½ teaspoon ground black pepper

Method

1. Heat up olive oil in the instant pot.
2. Then add diced garlic and saute it for 2 minutes.
3. After this, add broccoli florets, shredded cheese, heavy cream, and chicken broth.
4. Add ground black pepper and close the lid.
5. Cook the soup on manual mode (High pressure) for 3 minutes.
6. Then allow the natural pressure release for 5 minutes.

Nutritional info per serve: calories 285, fat 24.8, fiber 1.3, carbs 5.4, protein 11.5

Gumbo

Prep time: 10 minutes | **Cook time:** 15 minutes | **Yield:** 4 servings

Ingredients

- 2 chicken thighs, boneless, chopped
- 4 oz shrimps, peeled
- ½ bell pepper, chopped
- 3 oz sausages, chopped
- 1 celery stalk, chopped
- 1 cup beef broth
- 1 teaspoon tomato paste
- ½ teaspoon Cajun seasonings

Method

1. Heat up the instant pot on saute mode for 3 minutes.
2. Then add chicken thighs, shrimps, bell pepper, sausages, celery stalk, beef broth, tomato paste, and Cajun seasonings.
3. Gently mix up the ingredients and close the lid.
4. Cook the gumbo for 15 minutes on manual mode (high pressure).
5. Then make a quick pressure release and stir the meal well.

Nutritional info per serve: calories 261, fat 12.3, fiber 0.3, carbs 2.2, protein 33.2

Chicken Soup

Prep time: 10 minutes | **Cook time:** 20 minutes | **Yield:** 2 servings

Ingredients

- 8 oz chicken breast, skinless, boneless
- 2 cups of water
- 1 tablespoon
- scallions, diced
- 1 teaspoon salt
- 1 tablespoon fresh dill, chopped

Method

1. Pour water in the instant pot.
2. Chop the chicken breast and add it in the water.
3. Then add scallions, salt, and close the lid.
4. Cook the soup on manual mode (high pressure) for 20 minutes.
5. Then make a quick pressure release and ladle the soup in the bowls.
6. Top the soup with fresh dill.

Nutritional info per serve: calories 134, fat 2.9, fiber 0.3, carbs 1.1, protein 24.4

Taco Soup

Prep time: 15 minutes | **Cook time:** 20 minutes | **Yield:** 6 servings

Ingredients

- 1 cup ground beef
- 1 bell pepper, chopped
- 1 garlic clove, diced
- ½ cup crushed tomatoes
- 2 tablespoons cream cheese
- 4 cups beef broth
- 1 tablespoon coconut oil
- 1 teaspoon taco seasonings

Method

1. Heat up coconut oil in the instant pot on saute mode.
2. Then add ground beef and sprinkle it with taco seasonings. Stir well and cook the meat on saute mode for 5 minutes.
3. After this, add bell pepper, garlic clove, crushed tomatoes, cream cheese, and beef broth.
4. Close the lid and cook the soup on manual mode (high pressure) for 15 minutes.
5. Then allow the natural pressure release for 10 minutes and open the lid.
6. Ladle the soup.

Nutritional info per serve: calories 117, fat 7.1, fiber 1, carbs 4.4, protein 8.6

Tuscan Soup

Prep time: 15 minutes | **Cook time:** 13 minutes | **Yield:** 3 servings

Ingredients

- 1 bacon slice, chopped
- 2 oz scallions, diced
- ½ teaspoon garlic powder
- 6 oz Italian sausages, chopped
- ¼ cup cauliflower, chopped
- 3 cups chicken broth
- 1 cup kale, chopped
- ¼ cup heavy cream

Method

1. Heat up the instant pot on saute mode for 3 minutes.

2. Then add chopped bacon and cook it for 2 minutes on saute mode.

3. Stir it well and add scallions.

4. Add garlic powder, Italian sausages, and cauliflower.

5. Mix up the ingredients and cook them for 5 minutes on saute mode.

6. After this, add chicken broth, kale, and heavy cream.

7. Cook the soup on manual mode (high pressure) for 6 minutes. Then make a quick pressure release.

Nutritional info per serve: calories 324, fat 25.5, fiber 1.1, carbs 6.7, protein 16.7

Cabbage Soup

Prep time: 10 minutes | **Cook time:** 12 minutes | **Yield:** 3 servings

Ingredients

- ½ cup ground pork
- ½ cup white cabbage, shredded
- 2 cups chicken broth
- ½ teaspoon ground coriander
- ½ teaspoon salt
- 1 teaspoon butter
- ½ teaspoon chili flakes

Method

1. Melt the butter in the instant pot on saute mode.

2. Add cabbage and sprinkle it with ground coriander, salt, and chili flakes.

3. Add chicken broth and ground pork.

4. Close and seal the lid and cook the soup on manual mode (high pressure) for 12 minutes.

Nutritional info per serve: calories 350, fat 23.9, fiber 0.3, carbs 1.3, protein 30.2

Cauliflower Soup

Prep time: 15 minutes | **Cook time:** 6 minutes | **Yield:** 4 servings

Ingredients

- 2 cups cauliflower, chopped
- 1 cup coconut cream
- 2 cups beef broth
- 2 tablespoons fresh cilantro
- 3 oz Provolone cheese, chopped

Method

1. Put cauliflower, coconut cream, beef broth, cilantro, and cheese in the instant pot.

2. Cook the soup on manual (high pressure) for 6 minutes. Then allow the natural pressure release for 4 minutes.

3. Blend the soup with the help of the immersion blender.

Nutritional info per serve: calories 244, fat 20.7, fiber 2.6, carbs 6.9, protein 10.2

Cheeseburger Soup

Prep time: 10 minutes | **Cook time:** 11 minutes | **Yield:** 5 servings

Ingredients

- 1 cup ground pork
- 1 teaspoon mustard powder
- 4 cups beef broth
- 1 teaspoon cayenne pepper
- 1 teaspoon coconut oil
- ½ cup Monterey jack cheese, shredded
- 2 tablespoons cream cheese
- 3 tablespoons heavy cream

Method

1. In the mixing bowl, mix up ground pork, mustard powder, and cayenne pepper.

2. Then melt the coconut oil in the instant pot on saute mode.

3. Add the ground pork mixture and saute it for 6 minutes.

4. Then stir the mixture well and add cream cheese and heavy cream. Add beef broth and close the lid.

5. Cook the soup on manual mode (high pressure) for 5 minutes.

6. Then make a quick pressure release and ladle the soup in the bowls.

7. Top the soup with Monterey Jack cheese.

Nutritional info per serve: calories 316, fat 23.4, fiber 0.2, carbs 1.6, protein 23.4

Beef Stew

Prep time: 10 minutes | **Cook time:** 30 minutes | **Yield:** 4 servings

Ingredients

- ½ cup Brussel sprouts
- 4 cups of water
- 1 teaspoon tomato paste
- 12 oz beef sirloin, chopped
- 1 tablespoon sesame oil
- ½ teaspoon salt
- 1 bay leaf
- ½ teaspoon peppercorns

Method

1. Put all ingredients in the instant pot and close the lid.

2. Cook the stew on Manual mode (high pressure) for 30 minutes.

3. The cooked stew should have a very tender structure.

Nutritional info per serve: calories 195, fat 8.8, fiber 0.6, carbs 1.6, protein 26.3

Chili Verde Soup

Prep time: 10 minutes | **Cook time:** 25 minutes | **Yield:** 4 servings

Ingredients

- 2 oz chili Verde sauce
- ½ cup Cheddar cheese, shredded
- 5 cups chicken broth
- 1-pound chicken breast, skinless, boneless
- 1 tablespoon dried cilantro

Method

1. Put chicken breast and chicken broth in the instant pot.

2. Add cilantro, close and seal the lid.

3. Then cook the ingredients on manual (high pressure) for 15 minutes.

4. Make a quick pressure release and open the li.

5. Shred the chicken breast with the help of the fork.

6. Add dried cilantro and chili Verde sauce in the soup and cook it on saute mode for 10 minutes.

7. Then add dried cilantro and stir well.

Nutritional info per serve: calories 257, fat 10.2, fiber 0.2, carbs 4, protein 34.5

Curry Stew with Chicken

Prep time: 10 minutes | **Cook time:** 12 minutes | **Yield:** 4 servings

Ingredients

- 1 teaspoon curry paste
- 1 teaspoon grated lemon zest
- 4 oz leek, chopped
- 2 cups of water
- 1 tablespoon coconut cream
- 4 chicken thighs, skinless, boneless, chopped

Method

1. In the mixing bowl, mix up coconut cream, grated lemon zest, and curry paste.

2. Then mix up chopped chicken thighs and curry paste mixture.

3. Put the mixture in the instant pot and add leek and water.

4. Close the lid and cook the stew for 12 minutes on manual mode (high pressure).

5. Then make a quick pressure release and transfer the stew in the plates/bowls.

Nutritional info per serve: calories 145, fat 4.6, fiber 0.6, carbs 4.7, protein 20.4

Pepper Stuffing Soup

Prep time: 10 minutes | **Cook time:** 14 minutes | **Yield:** 4 servings

Ingredients

- 1 cup ground beef
- ½ cup cauliflower, shredded
- 1 teaspoon dried oregano
- ½ teaspoon salt
- 1 teaspoon tomato paste
- 1 teaspoon minced garlic
- 4 cups of water
- ¼ cup of coconut milk

Method

1. Put all ingredients in the instant pot bowl and stir well.

2. Then close and seal the lid.

3. Cook the soup on manual mode (high pressure) for 14 minutes.

4. When the time of cooking is finished, make a quick pressure release and open the lid.

Nutritional info per serve: calories 106, fat 7.7, fiber 0.9, carbs 2.2, protein 7.3

Chicken Paprikash

Prep time: 10 minutes | **Cook time:** 18 minutes | **Yield:** 4 servings

Ingredients

- 1 tablespoon ground paprika
- ¼ cup scallions, diced
- 1 bell pepper, chopped
- 4 chicken thighs, skinless
- 1 teaspoon coconut oil
- ½ teaspoon salt
- ½ teaspoon ground cumin
- 4 cups chicken broth

Method

1. Heat up coconut oil in the instant pot on Saute mode.
2. When the oil is melted. Add chicken thighs and cook them for 4 minutes from each side.
3. After this, sprinkle the chicken scallions, bell pepper, salt, and ground cumin. Gently mix up the ingredients. Add paprika.
4. Add chicken broth and close the lid.
5. Cook the paprikash for 10 minutes on Manual mode (high pressure). Then make a quick pressure release.

Nutritional info per serve: calories 343, fat 13.7, fiber 1.2, carbs 4.7, protein 47.8

Pork Stew

Prep time: 15 minutes | **Cook time:** 3 minutes | **Yield:** 6 servings

Ingredients

- ½ cup daikon, chopped
- 1 oz green onions, chopped
- 1-pound pork tenderloin, chopped
- 1 lemon slice
- 1 teaspoon ground black pepper
- 1 tablespoon butter
- 1 tablespoon heavy cream
- 3 cups of water

Method

1. Put all ingredients in the instant pot and mix up them with the help of the spatula.
2. Then close and seal the lid. Set manual mode (high pressure) and cook the stew for 20 minutes.
3. Allow the natural pressure release for 15 minutes.

Nutritional info per serve: calories 137, fat 5.5, fiber 0.3, carbs 0.9, protein 20.1

Italian Style Lamb Stew

Prep time: 10 minutes | **Cook time:** 52 minutes | **Yield:** 5 servings

Ingredients

- 1-pound lamb shank, chopped
- 1 teaspoon dried rosemary
- 1 turnip, chopped
- ½ teaspoon salt
- 1 teaspoon tomato paste
- 1 teaspoon olive oil
- 2 cups of water

Method

1. Heat up olive oil on saute mode for 2 minutes.
2. Then add turnip, chopped lamb shank, and dried rosemary. Saute the ingredients for 5 minutes.
3. After this, add water and tomato paste. Close the lid and cook the stew on saute mode for 45 minutes.

Nutritional info per serve: calories 185, fat 7.7, fiber 0.6, carbs 1.9, protein 25.8

Cheesy Cream Soup

Prep time: 15 minutes | **Cook time:** 20 minutes | **Yield:** 4 servings

Ingredients

- 3 tablespoons cream cheese
- 2 oz blue cheese, crumbled
- 2 cups white mushrooms, chopped
- 4 oz scallions, diced
- 4 cups chicken broth
- 1 teaspoon salt
- 1 teaspoon olive oil
- ½ teaspoon ground cumin

Method

1. Put cream cheese, mushrooms, scallions, chicken broth, olive oil, and ground cumin in the instant pot.
2. Close and seal the lid.
3. Cook the soup mixture for 20 minutes on manual mode (high pressure).
4. Then make a quick pressure release and open the lid.
5. Add salt and blend the soup with the help of the immersion blender.
6. Then ladle the soup in the bowls and top with blue cheese.

Nutritional info per serve: calories 142, fat 9.4, fiber 1.1, carbs 4.8, protein 10.1

Seafood Stew

Prep time: 10 minutes | **Cook time:** 20 minutes | **Yield:** 4 servings

Ingredients

- ½ teaspoon ground cumin
- ½ teaspoon ground paprika
- ½ teaspoon ground turmeric
- 8 oz cod, chopped
- ½ cup crushed tomatoes
- 1 teaspoon coconut oil
- ½ teaspoon sesame seeds

Method

1. Sprinkle the chopped cod with cumin, paprika, turmeric, and sesame seeds.

2. Then heat up coconut oil in the instant pot on saute mode.

3. Add cod and cook it for 2 minutes from each side.

4. Then add crushed tomatoes and close the lid.

5. Saute the stew for 15 minutes.

    Nutritional info per serve: calories 87, fat 1.9, fiber 1.2, carbs 3, protein 13.9

Okra and Beef Stew

Prep time: 15 minutes | **Cook time:** 25 minutes | **Yield:** 3 servings

Ingredients

- 6 oz okra, chopped
- 8 oz beef sirloin, chopped
- 1 cup of water
- ¼ cup coconut cream
- 1 teaspoon dried basil
- ¼ teaspoon cumin seeds
- 1 tablespoon avocado oil

Method

1. Sprinkle the beef sirloin with cumin seeds and dried basil and put in the instant pot.

2. Add avocado oil and roast the meat on saute mode for 5 minutes. Stir it occasionally.

3. Then add coconut cream, water, and okra.

4. Close the lid and cook the stew on manual mode (high pressure) for 25 minutes. Allow the natural pressure release for 10 minutes.

    Nutritional info per serve: calories 216, fat 10.2, fiber 2.5, carbs 5.7, protein 24.6

Chipotle Stew

Prep time: 15 minutes | **Cook time:** 10 minutes | **Yield:** 3 servings

Ingredients

- 2 chipotle chili in adobo sauce, chopped
- 1 oz fresh cilantro, chopped
- 9 oz chicken fillet, chopped
- 1 teaspoon ground paprika
- 2 tablespoons sesame seeds
- ¼ teaspoon salt
- 1 cup chicken broth

Method

1. In the mixing bowl mix up chipotle chili, cilantro, chicken fillet, ground paprika, sesame seeds, and salt.

2. Then transfer the ingredients in the instant pot and add chicken broth.

3. Cook the stew on manual mode (high pressure) for 10 minutes. Allow the natural pressure release for 10 minutes more.

    Nutritional info per serve: calories 230, fat 10.6, fiber 2.6, carbs 4.5, protein 27.6

Keto Chili

Prep time: 10 minutes | **Cook time:** 25 minutes | **Yield:** 2 servings

Ingredients

- ½ cup ground beef
- ½ teaspoon chili powder
- 1 teaspoon dried oregano
- ¼ cup crushed tomatoes
- 2 oz scallions, diced
- 1 teaspoon avocado oil
- ¼ cup of water

Method

1. Mix up ground beef, chili powder, dried oregano, and scallions.

2. Then add avocado oil and stir the mixture.

3. Transfer it in the instant pot and cook on saute mode for 10 minutes.

4. Add water and crushed tomatoes. Stir the ingredients with the help of the spatula until homogenous.

5. Close and seal the lid and cook the chili for 15 minutes on manual mode (high pressure). Then make a quick pressure release.

    Nutritional info per serve: calories 94, fat 4.6, fiber 2.4, carbs 5.6, protein 8

Pizza Soup

Prep time: 10 minutes | **Cook time:** 22 minutes | **Yield:** 3 servings

Ingredients

- ¼ cup cremini mushrooms, sliced
- 1 teaspoon tomato paste
- 4 oz Mozzarella, shredded
- ½ jalapeno pepper, sliced
- ½ teaspoon Italian seasoning
- 1 teaspoon coconut oil
- 5 oz Italian sausages, chopped
- 1 cup of water

Method

1. Melt the coconut oil in the instant pot on saute mode.
2. Add mushrooms and cook them for 10 minutes.
3. After this, add chopped sausages, Italian seasoning, sliced jalapeno, and tomato paste.
4. Mix up the ingredients well and add water.
5. Close and seal the lid and cook the soup on manual mode (high pressure) for 12 minutes.
6. Then make a quick pressure release and ladle the soup in the bowls. Top it with Mozzarella.

   Nutritional info per serve: calories 289, fat 23.2, fiber 0.2, carbs 2.5, protein 17.7

Lamb Soup

Prep time: 10 minutes | **Cook time:** 25 minutes | **Yield:** 4 servings

Ingredients

- ½ cup broccoli, roughly chopped
- 7 oz lamb fillet, chopped
- ¼ teaspoon ground cumin
- ¼ daikon, chopped
- 2 bell peppers, chopped
- 1 tablespoon avocado oil
- 5 cups beef broth

Method

1. Saute the lamb fillet with avocado oil in the instant pot for 5 minutes.
2. Then add broccoli, ground cumin, daikon, bell peppers, and beef broth.
3. Close and seal the lid.
4. Cook the soup on manual mode (high pressure) for 20 minutes.
5. Allow the natural pressure release.

   Nutritional info per serve: calories 169, fat 6, fiber 1.3, carbs 6.8, protein 21

Minestrone Soup

Prep time: 10 minutes | **Cook time:** 25 minutes | **Yield:** 4 servings

Ingredients

- 1 ½ cup ground pork
- ½ bell pepper, chopped
- 2 tablespoons chives, chopped
- 2 oz celery stalk, chopped
- 1 teaspoon butter
- 1 teaspoon Italian seasonings
- 4 cups chicken broth
- ½ cup mushrooms, sliced

Method

1. Heat up butter on the saute mode for 2 minutes.
2. Add bell pepper. Cook the vegetable for 5 minutes.
3. Then stir them well and add mushrooms, celery stalk, and Italian seasonings. Stir well and cook for 5 minutes more.
4. Add ground pork, chives, and chicken broth.
5. Close and seal the lid.
6. Cook the soup on manual mode (high pressure) for 15 minutes. Make a quick pressure release.

   Nutritional info per serve: calories 408, fat 27.2, fiber 0.6, carbs 3, protein 35.6

Chorizo Soup

Prep time: 10 minutes | **Cook time:** 17 minutes | **Yield:** 3 servings

Ingredients

- 8 oz chorizo, chopped
- 1 teaspoon tomato paste
- 4 oz scallions, diced
- 1 tablespoon dried
- cilantro
- ½ teaspoon chili powder
- 1 teaspoon avocado oil
- 2 cups beef broth

Method

1. Heat up avocado oil on saute mode for 1 minute.
2. Add chorizo and cook it for 6 minutes, stir it from time to time.
3. Then add scallions, tomato paste, cilantro, and chili powder. Stir well.
4. Add beef broth.
5. Close and seal the lid.
6. Cook the soup on manual mode (high pressure) for 10 minutes. Make a quick pressure release.

   Nutritional info per serve: calories 387, fat 30.2, fiber 1.3, carbs 5.5, protein 22.3

Red Feta Soup

Prep time: 10 minutes | **Cook time:** 25 minutes | **Yield:** 4 servings

Ingredients

- 1 cup broccoli, chopped
- 1 teaspoon tomato paste
- ½ cup coconut cream
- 4 cups beef broth
- 1 teaspoon chili flakes
- 6 oz feta, crumbled

Method

1. Put broccoli, tomato paste, coconut cream, and beef broth in the instant pot.
2. Add chili flakes and stir the mixture until it is red.
3. Then close and seal the lid and cook the soup for 8 minutes on manual mode (high pressure).
4. Then make a quick pressure release and open the lid.
5. Add feta cheese and saute the soup on saute mode for 5 minutes more.

   Nutritional info per serve: calories 229, fat 17.7, fiber 1.3, carbs 6.1, protein 12.3

"Ramen" Soup

Prep time: 10 minutes | **Cook time:** 15 minutes | **Yield:** 2 servings

Ingredients

- 1 zucchini, trimmed
- 2 cups chicken broth
- 2 eggs, boiled, peeled
- 1 tablespoon coconut aminos
- 5 oz beef loin, strips
- 1 teaspoon chili flakes
- 1 tablespoon chives, chopped
- ½ teaspoon salt

Method

1. Put the beef loin strips in the instant pot.
2. Add chili flakes, salt, and chicken broth.
3. Close and seal the lid. Cook the ingredients on manual mode (high pressure) for 15 minutes. Make a quick pressure release and open the lid.
4. Then make the s from zucchini with the help of the spiralizer and add them in the soup.
5. Add chives and coconut aminos.
6. Then ladle the soup in the bowls and top with halved eggs.

   Nutritional info per serve: calories 254, fat 11.8, fiber 1.1, carbs 6.2, protein 30.6

Beef Tagine

Prep time: 15 minutes | **Cook time:** 25 minutes | **Yield:** 6 servings

Ingredients

- 1-pound beef fillet, chopped
- 1 eggplant, chopped
- 6 oz scallions, chopped
- 1 teaspoon ground
- allspices
- 1 teaspoon Erythritol
- 1 teaspoon coconut oil
- 4 cups beef broth

Method

1. Put all ingredients in the instant pot.
2. Close and seal the lid.
3. Cook the meal on manual mode (high pressure) for 25 minutes.
4. Then allow the natural pressure release for 15 minutes.

   Nutritional info per serve: calories 146, fat 5.3, fiber 3.5, carbs 8.8, protein 16.7

Leek Soup

Prep time: 10 minutes | **Cook time:** 15 minutes | **Yield:** 4 servings

Ingredients

- 7 oz leek, chopped
- 2 oz Monterey Jack cheese, shredded
- 1 teaspoon Italian
- seasonings
- ½ teaspoon salt
- 4 tablespoons butter
- 2 cups chicken broth

Method

1. Heat up butter in the instant pot for 4 minutes.
2. Then add chopped leek, salt, and Italian seasonings.
3. Cook the leek on saute mode for 5 minutes. Stir the vegetables from time to time.
4. After this, add chicken broth and close the lid.
5. Cook the soup on saute mode for 10 minutes.
6. Then add shredded cheese and stir it till the cheese is melted.
7. The soup is cooked.

   Nutritional info per serve: calories 208, fat 17, fiber 0.9, carbs 7.7, protein 6.8

Asparagus Soup

Prep time: 10 minutes | **Cook time:** 17 minutes | **Yield:** 4 servings

Ingredients

- 1 cup asparagus, chopped
- 2 cups of coconut milk
- 1 teaspoon salt
- ½ teaspoon cayenne pepper
- 3 oz scallions, diced
- 1 teaspoon olive oil

Method

1. Saute the chopped asparagus, scallions, and olive oil in the instant pot for 7 minutes.
2. Then stir the vegetables well and add cayenne pepper, salt, and coconut milk
3. Cook the soup on manual mode (high pressure) for 10 minutes.
4. After this, make a quick pressure release and open the lid.
5. Blend the soup until you get the creamy texture.

Nutritional info per serve: calories 300, fat 29.9, fiber 4, carbs 9.6, protein 3.9

Steak Soup

Prep time: 10 minutes | **Cook time:** 40 minutes | **Yield:** 5 servings

Ingredients

- 5 oz scallions, diced
- 1 tablespoon coconut oil
- 1 oz daikon, diced
- 1-pound beef round steak, chopped
- 1 teaspoon dried thyme
- 5 cups of water
- ½ teaspoon ground black pepper

Method

1. Heat up coconut oil on saute mode for 2 minutes.
2. Add daikon and scallions.
3. After this, stir them well and add chopped beef steak, thyme, and ground black pepper.
4. Saute the ingredients for 5 minutes more and then add water.
5. Close and seal the lid.
6. Cook the soup on manual mode (high pressure) for 35 minutes. Make a quick pressure release.

Nutritional info per serve: calories 232, fat 11, fiber 0.9, carbs 2.5, protein 29.5

Meat Spinach Stew

Prep time: 20 minutes | **Cook time:** 30 minutes | **Yield:** 4 servings

Ingredients

- 2 cups spinach, chopped
- 1-pound beef sirloin, chopped
- 1 teaspoon allspices
- 3 cups chicken broth
- 1 cup of coconut milk
- 1 teaspoon coconut aminos

Method

1. Put all ingredients in the instant pot.
2. Close and seal the lid.
3. After this, set the manual mode (high pressure) and cook the stew for 30 minutes.
4. When the cooking time is finished, allow the natural pressure release for 10 minutes.
5. Stir the stew gently before serving.

Nutritional info per serve: calories 383, fat 22.2, fiber 1.8, carbs 5.1, protein 39.9

Curry Kale Soup

Prep time: 10 minutes | **Cook time:** 15 minutes | **Yield:** 3 servings

Ingredients

- 2 cups kale
- 1 tablespoon fresh cilantro
- 1 teaspoon curry paste
- ½ cup heavy cream
- ½ cup ground chicken
- 1 teaspoon almond butter
- ½ teaspoon salt
- 1 cup chicken stock

Method

1. Blend the kale until smooth and put it in the instant pot.
2. Add cilantro, almond butter, and ground chicken. Saute the mixture for 5 minutes.
3. Meanwhile, in the shallow bowl, mix up curry paste and heavy cream. When the liquid is smooth, pour it in the instant pot.
4. Add chicken stock and salt, and close the lid.
5. Cook the soup on manual (high pressure) for 10 minutes. Make a quick pressure release.

Nutritional info per serve: calories 183, fat 13.3, fiber 1.2, carbs 7, protein 9.9

Tomatillos Fish Stew

Prep time: 15 minutes | **Cook time:** 12 minutes | **Yield:** 2 servings

Ingredients

- 2 tomatillos, chopped
- 10 oz salmon fillet, chopped
- 1 teaspoon ground paprika
- ½ teaspoon ground turmeric
- 1 cup coconut cream
- ½ teaspoon salt

Method

1. Put all ingredients in the instant pot.
2. Close and seal the lid.
3. Cook the fish stew on manual mode (high pressure) for 12 minutes.
4. Then allow the natural pressure release for 10 minutes.

    Nutritional info per serve: calories 479, fat 37.9, fiber 3.8, carbs 9.6, protein 30.8

Jalapeno Soup

Prep time: 10 minutes | **Cook time:** 10 minutes | **Yield:** 4 servings

Ingredients

- 2 jalapeno peppers, sliced
- 3 oz pancetta, chopped
- ½ cup heavy cream
- 2 cups of water
- ½ cup Monterey jack cheese, shredded
- ½ teaspoon garlic powder
- 1 teaspoon coconut oil
- ½ teaspoon smoked paprika

Method

1. Toss pancetta in the instant pot, add coconut oil and cook it for 4 minutes on saute mode. Stir it from time to time.
2. After this, add sliced jalapenos, garlic powder, and smoked paprika.
3. Stir the ingredients for 1 minute.
4. Add heavy cream and water.
5. Then add Monterey Jack cheese and stir the soup well.
6. Close and seal the lid; cook the soup for 5 minutes on manual mode (high pressure); make a quick pressure release.

    Nutritional info per serve: calories 234, fat 20, fiber 0.4, carbs 1.7, protein 11.8

Cream of Mushrooms Soup

Prep time: 10 minutes | **Cook time:** 35 minutes | **Yield:** 6 servings

Ingredients

- 3 cups cremini mushrooms, sliced
- 1 cup of coconut milk
- 1 tablespoon almond flour
- 1 teaspoon salt
- 1 teaspoon ground black pepper
- 4 cups chicken broth
- 3 tablespoons butter

Method

1. Melt the butter on saute mode.
2. Add cremini mushrooms and saute them for 10 minutes. Stir them with the help of the spatula from time to time.
3. After this, in the bowl mix up salt, almond flour, and ground black pepper. Add coconut milk and stir the liquid.
4. Pour the liquid over the mushrooms.
5. Add chicken broth. Close and seal the lid.
6. Cook the soup on saute mode for 25 minutes.

    Nutritional info per serve: calories 206, fat 18.6, fiber 1.7, carbs 5.5, protein 6.2

Turmeric Rutabaga Soup

Prep time: 15 minutes | **Cook time:** 15 minutes | **Yield:** 5 servings

Ingredients

- 3 turnips, chopped
- 1 teaspoon ginger paste
- 2 oz celery, chopped
- 1 teaspoon ground turmeric
- 1 teaspoon minced garlic
- 2 cups of coconut milk
- 1 cup beef broth
- 2 oz bell pepper, chopped

Method

1. Place all ingredients in the instant pot and stir them gently.
2. Then close and seal the lid; set manual mode (high pressure) and cook the soup for 15 minutes.
3. Then allow the natural pressure release for 10 minutes and ladle the soup into the serving bowls.

    Nutritional info per serve: calories 255, fat 23.2, fiber 3.6, carbs 11.4, protein 4

Bok Choy Soup

Prep time: 5 minutes | **Cook time:** 2 minutes | **Yield:** 1 serving

Ingredients

- 1 bok choy stalk, chopped
- ¼ teaspoon nutritional yeast
- ½ teaspoon onion powder
- ¼ teaspoon chili flakes
- 1 cup chicken broth

Method

1. Put all ingredients from the list above in the instant pot.

2. Close and seal the lid and cook the soup on manual (high pressure) for 2 minutes.

3. Make a quick pressure release.

Nutritional info per serve: calories 58 fat 1.7, fiber 1.3, carbs 4.5, protein 6.9

Garden Soup

Prep time: 20 minutes | **Cook time:** 29 minutes | **Yield:** 5 servings

Ingredients

- ½ cup cauliflower florets
- 1 cup kale, chopped
- 1 garlic clove, diced
- 1 tablespoon olive oil
- 1 1 teaspoon sea salt
- 6 cups beef broth
- 2 tablespoons chives, chopped

Method

1. Heat up olive oil in the instant pot on saute mode for 2 minutes and add clove.

2. Cook the vegetables for 2 minutes and stir well.

3. Add kale, cauliflower, sea salt, chives, and beef broth.

4. Close and seal the lid.

5. Cook the soup on manual mode (high pressure) for 5 minutes.

6. Then make a quick pressure release and open the lid.

7. Ladle the soup into the bowls.

Nutritional info per serve: calories 80, fat 4.5, fiber 0.5, carbs 2.3, protein 6.5

Shirataki Noodle Soup

Prep time: 25 minutes | **Cook time:** 15 minutes | **Yield:** 2 servings

Ingredients

- 2 oz shirataki noodles
- 2 cups of water
- 6 oz chicken fillet, chopped
- 1 teaspoon salt
- 1 tablespoon coconut aminos

Method

1. Pour water in the instant pot bowl.

2. Add salt and chopped chicken fillet. Close and seal the lid.

3. Cook the ingredients on manual mode (high pressure) for 15 minutes. Allow the natural pressure release for 10 minutes.

4. After this, add shirataki noodles and coconut aminos.

5. Leave the soup for 10 minutes to rest.

Nutritional info per serve: calories 175, fat 6.3, fiber 3, carbs 1.5, protein 24.8

Flu Soup

Prep time: 10 minutes | **Cook time:** 15 minutes | **Yield:** 4 servings

Ingredients

- 1 cup mushrooms, chopped
- 1 cup spinach, chopped
- 3 oz scallions, diced
- 2 oz Cheddar cheese, shredded
- 1 teaspoon cayenne pepper
- 1 cup organic almond milk
- 2 cups chicken broth
- ½ teaspoon salt

Method

1. Put all ingredients in the instant pot and close the lid.

2. Set the manual mode (high pressure) and cook the soup for 15 minutes.

3. Make a quick pressure release.

4. Blend the soup with the help of the immersion blender.

5. When the soup will get smooth texture – it is cooked.

Nutritional info per serve: calories 228, fat 19.9, fiber 2.3, carbs 6.6, protein 8.5

Vegan Cream Soup

Prep time: 5 minutes | **Cook time:** 8 minutes | **Yield:** 2 servings

Ingredients

- 1 cup of coconut milk
- 1 teaspoon coconut oil
- ½ teaspoon paprika
- 2 cups cauliflower, chopped
- 1 teaspoon salt
- 1 teaspoon chives, chopped

Method

1. Mix up all ingredients in the instant pot.
2. Set the "Manual" mode and turn on the timer on 8 minutes (High pressure).
3. When the time is finished, make a quick pressure release.
4. Use the hand blender to make the cream soup smooth.

Nutritional info per serve: calories 322, fat 31.1, fiber 5.4, carbs 12.3, protein 4.8

Bacon Soup

Prep time: 10 minutes | **Cook time:** 20 minutes | **Yield:** 4 servings

Ingredients

- 3 oz bacon, chopped
- 1 cup cheddar cheese, shredded
- 1 tablespoon scallions, chopped
- 3 cups beef broth
- 1 cup of coconut milk
- 1 teaspoon curry powder

Method

1. Heat up the instant pot on saute mode for 3 minutes and add bacon.
2. Cook it for 5 minutes. Stir it from time to time.
3. Then add scallions and curry powder. Cook the ingredients for 5 minutes more. Stir them from time to time.
4. After this, add coconut milk and beef broth.
5. Add cheddar cheese and stir the soup well.
6. Cook it on manual mode (high pressure) for 10 minutes. Make a quick pressure release.
7. Mix up the soup well before serving.

Nutritional info per serve: calories 398, fat 33.6, fiber 1.5, carbs 5.1, protein 20

Paprika Zucchini Soup

Prep time: 10 minutes | **Cook time:** 1 minute | **Yield:** 2 servings

Ingredients

- 1 zucchini, grated
- 1 teaspoon ground paprika
- ½ teaspoon cayenne pepper
- ½ cup of coconut milk
- 1 cup beef broth
- 1 tablespoon dried cilantro
- 1 oz Parmesan, grated

Method

1. Put the grated zucchini, paprika, cayenne pepper, coconut milk, beef broth, and dried cilantro in the instant pot.
2. Close and seal the lid.
3. Cook the soup on manual (high pressure) for 1 minute. Make a quick pressure release.
4. Ladle the soup in the serving bowls and top with parmesan.

Nutritional info per serve: calories 223, fat 18.4, fiber 2.9, carbs 8.4, protein 9.7

Pancetta Chowder

Prep time: 5 minutes | **Cook time:** 8 minutes | **Yield:** 3 servings

Ingredients

- 1 cup of coconut milk
- 4 oz pancetta, chopped, fried
- 1 oz celery stalk, chopped
- ¼ teaspoon salt
- 1 teaspoon ground paprika

Method

1. Pour the coconut milk in the instant pot bowl.
2. Add celery stalk in the instant pot bowl too.
3. After this, add salt and paprika.
4. Lock the instant pot lid and seal it.
5. Press the "Manual" mode (High pressure) and set the timer for 3 minutes.
6. Then make naturally pressure release for 5 minutes.
7. Top the cooked chowder with fried pancetta.

Nutritional info per serve: calories 392, fat 35, fiber 2.2, carbs 5.6, protein 16

Egg Drop Soup

Prep time: 5 minutes | **Cook time:** 10 minutes | **Yield:** 4 servings

Ingredients

- 4 cups chicken broth
- 2 tablespoons fresh dill, chopped
- 2 eggs, beaten
- 1 teaspoon salt

Method

1. Pour chicken broth in the instant pot.
2. Add salt and bring it to boil on Saute mode.
3. Then add beaten eggs and stir the liquid well.
4. Add dill and saute it for 5 minutes.
5. The soup is cooked.

   Nutritional info per serve: calories 74, fat 3.6, fiber 0.2, carbs 2, protein 7.9

Buffalo Style Soup

Prep time: 7 minutes | **Cook time:** 10 minutes | **Yield:** 2 servings

Ingredients

- 6 oz chicken, cooked
- 2 oz Mozzarella, shredded
- 4 tablespoons coconut milk
- ¼ teaspoon white pepper
- ¾ teaspoon salt
- 2 tablespoons keto Buffalo sauce
- 1 oz celery stalk, chopped
- 1 cup of water

Method

1. Place the chopped celery stalk, water, salt, white pepper, coconut milk, and Mozzarella in the instant pot. Stir it gently.
2. Set the "Manual" mode (High pressure) and turn on the timer for 7 minutes.
3. Shred the cooked chicken and combine it together with Buffalo Sauce.
4. Make quick pressure release and transfer the soup on the bowls.
5. Add shredded chicken and stir it.

   Nutritional info per serve: calories 287, fat 14.8, fiber 1.5, carbs 4.3, protein 33.5

Cordon Blue Soup

Prep time: 15 minutes | **Cook time:** 6 minutes | **Yield:** 4 servings

Ingredients

- 4 cups chicken broth
- 7 oz ham, chopped
- 3 oz Mozzarella cheese, shredded
- 1 teaspoon ground black pepper
- ½ teaspoon salt
- 2 tablespoons ricotta cheese
- 2 oz scallions, chopped

Method

1. Put all ingredients in the instant pot bowl and stir gently.
2. Close and seal the lid; cook the soup on manual mode (high pressure) for 6 minutes.
3. Then allow the natural pressure release for 10 minutes and ladle the soup into the bowls.

   Nutritional info per serve: calories 196, fat 10.1, fiber 1.2, carbs 5.3, protein 20.3

Beef & Lamb

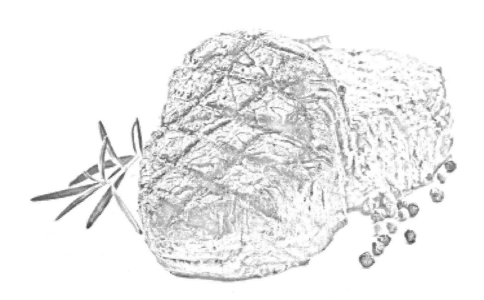

Beef Pot Roast

Prep time: 20 minutes | **Cook time:** 40 minutes | **Yield:** 5 servings

Ingredients

- 1-pound beef chuck roast, chopped
- 1 teaspoon salt
- 4 tablespoon apple cider vinegar
- ¾ teaspoon xanthan gum
- 1 cup beef broth
- 1 teaspoon olive oil

Method

1. Sprinkle the beef with olive oil and salt.
2. Then put it in the instant pot and add beef broth, apple cider vinegar, and xanthan gum. Stir the ingredients gently with the help of the spoon. Close and seal the lid.
3. Cook the meal on manual mode (high pressure) for 40 minutes.
4. Then allow the natural pressure release for 10 minutes.

Nutritional info per serve: calories 350, fat 26.4, fiber 0.7, carbs 1, protein 24.7

Mongolian Beef

Prep time: 10 minutes | **Cook time:** 45 minutes | **Yield:** 4 servings

Ingredients

- 1 tablespoon coconut aminos
- ¼ teaspoon garlic, minced
- 1 teaspoon Erythritol
- 1 teaspoon sesame oil
- ¼ teaspoon ground ginger
- 1-pound flank steak
- ¼ cup of water

Method

1. In the mixing bowl mix up coconut aminos, minced garlic, Erythritol, and ground ginger.
2. Slice the flank steak and mix it up with coconut aminos mixture.
3. Heat up sesame oil on saute mode for 1 minute and add sliced flank steal
4. Cook it for 10 minutes on saute mode. Stir it from time to time.
5. Then add water and close the lid.
6. Cook the beef on saute mode for 35 minutes.

Nutritional info per serve: calories 234, fat 10.6, fiber 0, carbs 0.9, protein 31.6

Thyme Beef Brisket

Prep time: 10 minutes | **Cook time:** 25 minutes | **Yield:** 3 servings

Ingredients

- 1 teaspoon dried thyme
- 12 oz beef brisket, chopped
- ½ cup of water
- ½ teaspoon salt
- 1 teaspoon coconut oil

Method

1. Sprinkle the beef brisket with salt and dried thyme.
2. Then melt the coconut oil in the instant pot on saute mode and add beef brisket.
3. Add water and close the lid.
4. Cook the meat on manual mode (high pressure) for 25 minutes.
5. Then allow the natural pressure release for 10 minutes.

Nutritional info per serve: calories 225, fat 8.6, fiber 0.1, carbs 0.2, protein 34.4

Goulash

Prep time: 10 minutes | **Cook time:** 35 minutes | **Yield:** 4 servings

Ingredients

- 1-pound beef sirloin, chopped
- 1 bell pepper, chopped
- 2 celery stalks, chopped
- 1 teaspoon coconut oil
- 1 teaspoon chili flakes
- 1 cup of water

Method

1. Put the coconut oil and chopped beef sirloin in the instant pot.
2. Cook it on sauté mode for 5 minutes. Stir it with the help of a spatula and add chili flakes.
3. Then add celery stalk and water.
4. Add bell pepper. Close and seal the lid.
5. Cook the goulash for 30 minutes on manual mode (high pressure). Make a quick pressure release.

Nutritional info per serve: calories 231, fat 8.3, fiber 0.6, carbs 2.5, protein 34.8

Beef Pot Round Steak

Prep time: 10 minutes | **Cook time:** 25 minutes | **Yield:** 2 servings

Ingredients

- 2 pork round steaks
- 2 tablespoons avocado oil
- 1 teaspoon white pepper
- ½ teaspoon salt
- 1 teaspoon cayenne pepper
- 1 cup of water

Method

1. Rub the round steaks with avocado oil, white pepper, salt, and cayenne pepper.

2. Then wrap it in the foil.

3. Pour water and insert the rack in the instant pot.

4. Then put the wrapped steaks on the rack. Close and seal the lid.

5. Cook the steaks on manual mode (high pressure) for 25 minutes.

6. When the time is over, make a quick pressure release and open the lid.

7. Remove the steaks from the foil.

Nutritional info per serve: calories 334, fat 21, fiber 2.1, carbs 8, protein 29.4

Steak Bites

Prep time: 10 minutes | **Cook time:** 35 minutes | **Yield:** 6 servings

Ingredients

- 1-pound beef sirloin steak
- 3 tablespoons coconut aminos
- 1 teaspoon red
- pepper flakes
- ½ teaspoon minced garlic
- 3 tablespoons sesame oil

Method

1. Cut the beef sirloin steak on small cubes (bites) and sprinkle them with coconut aminos, red pepper flakes, minced garlic, and sesame oil.

2. Leave the meat for 10 minutes to marinate.

3. Then heat up the instant pot on saute mode.

4. Add the beef bites and close the lid.

5. Cook the meal for 35 minutes on saute mode. Stir it every 5 minutes to avoid burning.

Nutritional info per serve: calories 209, fat 11.6, fiber 0.1, carbs 1.8, protein 23

Hibachi Steak

Prep time: 10 minutes | **Cook time:** 10 minutes | **Yield:** 4 servings

Ingredients

- 1-pound beef sirloin, roughly chopped
- 1 teaspoon ground ginger
- ¼ teaspoon garlic powder
- ¼ cup cremini
- mushrooms, sliced
- 2 tablespoons apple cider vinegar
- 1 tablespoon avocado oil
- ¼ cup of water

Method

1. Mix up beef sirloin, ground ginger, garlic powder, apple cider vinegar, mushrooms, and avocado oil.

2. Transfer the ingredients in the instant pot. Add water.

3. Close and seal the lid and cook the meal on manual mode (high pressure) for 10 minutes. Allow the natural pressure release for 10 minutes.

Nutritional info per serve: calories 220, fat 7.5, fiber 0.3, carbs 0.9, protein 34.6

Beef Burgundy

Prep time: 15 minutes | **Cook time:** 35 minutes | **Yield:** 6 servings

Ingredients

- 3 oz bacon, chopped
- 1-pound beef tenderloin, chopped
- 1 teaspoon tomato paste
- ¼ cup apple cider vinegar
- 1 cup beef broth
- ¼ teaspoon xanthan gum
- ¼ teaspoon ground coriander
- 1 teaspoon dried oregano

Method

1. Put the bacon in the instant pot and cook it for 5 minutes on saute mode.

2. Stir the bacon with the help of the spatula every 1 minute.

3. Then add chopped beef tenderloin, apple cider vinegar, xanthan gum, ground coriander, and dried oregano.

4. Then add tomato paste and mix up the meat mixture.

5. Add beef broth and close the lid.

6. Cook the meal on manual mode (high pressure) for 30 minutes. Make a quick pressure release.

Nutritional info per serve: calories 245, fat 13.1, fiber 0.7, carbs 1.3, protein 28

Beef Gyros Stuffing

Prep time: 10 minutes | **Cook time:** 22 minutes | **Yield:** 2 servings

Ingredients

- 5 oz beef chuck, sliced
- 1 teaspoon chives, chopped
- ¾ cup beef broth
- 1 teaspoon coconut aminos
- ½ teaspoon olive oil
- ¼ teaspoon Italian seasonings

Method

1. Put the sliced beef chuck in the instant pot.
2. Add chives, beef broth, coconut aminos, olive oil, and Italian seasonings.
3. Cook the beef gyros stuffing for 22 minutes on saute mode. Mix it up every 5 minutes.

   Nutritional info per serve: calories 160, fat 6.3, fiber 0, carbs 0.9, protein 23.3

Butter Beef

Prep time: 10 minutes | **Cook time:** 7 hours | **Yield:** 4 servings

Ingredients

- 1-pound beef steak
- ½ cup butter, softened
- 1 teaspoon ground nutmeg
- ½ teaspoon salt

Method

1. Heat up butter in the instant pot on saute mode.
2. When the butter is melted, add beef steak, ground nutmeg, and salt.
3. Close the lid and cook the meat on slow cook mode for 7 hours.

   Nutritional info per serve: calories 417, fat 30.3, fiber 0.1, carbs 0.3, protein 34.7

Lamb Masala

Prep time: 10 minutes | **Cook time:** 25 minutes | **Yield:** 3 servings

Ingredients

- 12 oz lamb sirloin, sliced
- 1 tablespoon garam masala
- 1 tablespoon lemon juice
- 1 tablespoon olive oil
- ¼ cup coconut cream

Method

1. Sprinkle the sliced lamb sirloin with garam masala, lemon juice, olive oil, and coconut cream. Mix up the meat mixture well and transfer it in the instant pot.
2. Cook it on saute mode for 25 minutes.
3. Stir the lamb masala every 5 minutes.

   Nutritional info per serve: calories 319, fat 19.9, fiber 0.5, carbs 1.2, protein 32.7

Lamb Kleftiko

Prep time: 25 minutes | **Cook time:** 50 minutes | **Yield:** 6 servings

Ingredients

- 1-pound lamb shoulder, chopped
- ½ cup turnip, chopped
- 1 tablespoon lemon juice
- ½ teaspoon lemon
- zest, grated
- ¼ cup apple cider vinegar
- ½ cup chicken broth
- ½ teaspoon fresh thyme

Method

1. In the mixing bowl, mix up lemon juice, lemon zest, apple cider vinegar, chicken broth, and thyme.
2. Then put the lamb shoulder in the instant pot.
3. Add lemon juice mixture and turnip.
4. Close and seal the lid.
5. Cook the meal on manual mode (high pressure) for 50 minutes.
6. When the time is over, allow the natural pressure release for 20 minutes.

   Nutritional info per serve: calories 150, fat 5.7, fiber 0.2, carbs 1, protein 21.8

Greek Style Leg of Lamb

Prep time: 10 minutes | **Cook time:** 50 minutes | **Yield:** 4 servings

Ingredients

- 1-pound leg of lamb
- 2 garlic cloves, peeled
- 1 teaspoon paprika powder
- ½ teaspoon dried
- thyme
- ¼ teaspoon cumin seeds
- ¼ cup of water
- 1 tablespoon butter

Method

1. Rub the leg of lamb with paprika powder, dried thyme, and cumin seeds.
2. Then gently brush it with softened butter and transfer in the instant pot.
3. Add garlic cloves and water.
4. Close and seal the lid.
5. Cook the meal on manual mode (high pressure) for 50 minutes. Make a quick pressure release.

   Nutritional info per serve: calories 239, fat 11.2, fiber 0.1, carbs 0.6, protein 32

Lamb Curry

Prep time: 10 minutes | **Cook time:** 30 minutes | **Yield:** 4 servings

Ingredients

- 1-pound lamb shoulder, chopped
- 1 teaspoon curry paste
- 2 tablespoons coconut cream
- ¼ teaspoon chili powder
- 1 tablespoon fresh cilantro, chopped
- ½ cup heavy cream

Method

1. In the shallow bowl mix up curry paste and coconut cream.
2. Add chili powder and chopped lamb shoulder. Coat the meat in the curry mixture well.
3. Then transfer the meat and all remaining curry paste mixture in the instant pot.
4. Add cilantro and heavy cream.
5. Close and seal the lid and cook the meal for 30 minutes on manual mode (high pressure). Make a quick pressure release.

Nutritional info per serve: calories 289, fat 16.4, fiber 0.2, carbs 1.3, protein 32.4

Persian Lamb

Prep time: 10 minutes | **Cook time:** 40 minutes | **Yield:** 4 servings

Ingredients

- ¼ cup pomegranate juice
- ¼ teaspoon ground coriander
- 1 oz scallions, chopped
- 1-pound lamb fillet, chopped
- 1 teaspoon coconut oil
- ½ cup of water

Method

1. Heat up the coconut oil on saute mode for 2 minutes.
2. Add lamb fillet and cook it on saute mode for 5 minutes.
3. Then stir it well and add scallions, ground coriander, and pomegranate juice.
4. Add water, close and seal the lid.
5. Cook the meat for 32 minutes on manual mode (high pressure). Make a quick pressure release.

Nutritional info per serve: calories 232, fat 9.5, fiber 0.2, carbs 2.8, protein 32

Lamb Roast

Prep time: 10 minutes | **Cook time:** 25 minutes | **Yield:** 3 servings

Ingredients

- 14 oz leg of lamb, roughly chopped
- 1 teaspoon ground black pepper
- 1 teaspoon dried
- thyme
- 1 tablespoon sesame oil
- ¼ cup beef broth
- ½ cup of water

Method

1. Sprinkle the meat with ground black pepper, thyme, and sesame oil.
2. Then put it in the instant pot, add beef broth and water.
3. Close and seal the lid.
4. Cook the meal on manual mode (high pressure) for 25 minutes.
5. When the time is finished, make a quick pressure release.

Nutritional info per serve: calories 292, fat 14.4, fiber 0.3, carbs 0.7, protein 37.7

Lamb Bhuna

Prep time: 15 minutes | **Cook time:** 20 minutes | **Yield:** 2 servings

Ingredients

- ¼ teaspoon minced ginger
- 2 oz scallions, chopped
- 1 teaspoon coconut oil
- 10 oz lamb fillet,
- chopped
- ¼ teaspoon garlic paste
- ¼ cup crushed tomatoes
- ¼ cup of water

Method

1. Put the coconut oil, minced ginger, garlic paste, and crushed tomatoes in the instant pot.
2. Saute the mixture for 10 minutes.
3. Then stir it well and add scallions, chopped lamb fillet, and water.
4. Cook the lamb bhuna for 10 minutes on manual mode (high pressure).
5. When the time is finished, allow the natural pressure release for 15 minutes.

Nutritional info per serve: calories 306, fat 12.7, fiber 1.8, carbs 4.9, protein 41.1

Beef Vindaloo

Prep time: 15 minutes | **Cook time:** 15 minutes | **Yield:** 2 servings

Ingredients

- ½ serrano pepper, chopped
- ¼ teaspoon cumin seeds
- 9 oz beef clod, chopped
- ¼ teaspoon salt
- ¼ teaspoon ground paprika
- ¼ teaspoon minced ginger
- 1 cup of water
- ¼ teaspoon cayenne pepper

Method

1. Put serrano pepper, cumin seeds, salt, ground paprika, minced ginger, cayenne pepper, and water in the blender.
2. Blend the mixture till you get a smooth texture.
3. Then transfer it in the bowl and add chopped beef clod. Coat the meat in the blended mixture well.
4. Transfer the ingredients in the instant pot and close the lid.
5. Cook the meal on manual mode (high pressure) for 15 minutes.
6. Then allow the natural pressure release for 10 minutes.

Nutritional info per serve: calories 376, fat 27.4, fiber 0.3, carbs 0.7, protein 29.9

Rogan Josh

Prep time: 5 minutes | **Cook time:** 15 minutes | **Yield:** 4 servings

Ingredients

- 1 teaspoon ground cardamom
- ½ teaspoon coriander powder
- ½ teaspoon ground turmeric
- ¼ teaspoon chili powder
- 1-pound lamb shoulder, boneless, chopped
- ½ cup organic almond milk
- 1 teaspoon tomato paste
- 1 teaspoon coconut oil

Method

1. Put all ingredients in the instant pot and mix up.
2. Then close and seal the lid.
3. Cook the meal in manual mode for 15 minutes. Make a quick pressure release.
4. Open the lid and stir the cooked Rogan Josh well. Top the cooked meal with chopped cilantro, if desired.

Nutritional info per serve: calories 232, fat 9.9, fiber 0.3, carbs 1.9, protein 32.1

Icelandic Lamb

Prep time: 5 minutes | **Cook time:** 45 minutes | **Yield:** 4 servings

Ingredients

- 3 oz celery ribs, chopped
- ¼ cup scallions, chopped
- 4 oz turnip, chopped
- 1 teaspoon tomato paste
- ½ teaspoon ground black pepper
- ½ teaspoon salt
- 4 cups of water
- 12 oz lamb fillet, chopped

Method

1. Put all ingredients in the instant pot and stir well until the tomato paste is dissolved.
2. Then close and seal the lid.
3. Cook the lamb on manual (high pressure) for 45 minutes.
4. Then make the quick pressure release, open the lid, and mix up the lamb well.

Nutritional info per serve: calories 173, fat 6.3, fiber 1.1, carbs 3.3, protein 24.5

Harissa Lamb Shoulder

Prep time: 30 minutes | **Cook time:** 40 minutes | **Yield:** 4 servings

Ingredients

- 16 oz lamb shoulder
- 1 tablespoon harissa
- 2 tablespoons sesame oil
- 2 cups of water
- 1 teaspoon dried thyme
- ½ teaspoon salt

Method

1. In the shallow bowl mix up harissa and dried thyme.
2. Then rub the lamb shoulder with the spice mixture and brush with sesame oil.
3. Heat up the instant pot on saute mode for 2 minutes and put the lamb shoulder inside.
4. Cook the meat for 3 minutes from each side. Add water.
5. Close and seal the lid.
6. Cook it on manual mode (high pressure) for 40 minutes.
7. When the cooking time is finished, allow the natural pressure release for 25 minutes.

Nutritional info per serve: calories 284, fat 15.8, fiber 0.1, carbs 1.7, protein 32.1

Kofta Curry

Prep time: 15 minutes | **Cook time:** 20 minutes | **Yield:** 4 servings

Ingredients

- 1-pound ground lamb
- 1 tablespoon curry powder
- 1/3 cup coconut cream
- 4 oz scallions, chopped
- 1 cup chicken broth
- 1 tablespoon dried cilantro
- ½ teaspoon chili flakes
- 1 tablespoon coconut oil

Method

1. In the mixing bowl, mix up ½ tablespoon of curry powder, scallions, and ground lamb.
2. Add chili flakes and dried cilantro. Stir the mixture until homogenous and make the medium size koftas (meatballs).
3. Then heat up the coconut oil until it is melted (saute mode).
4. Put the koftas in the hot oil and cook them for 2 minutes from each side.
5. Then mix up coconut cream and remaining curry powder. Add chicken broth and pour the liquid over the koftas.
6. Cook the meal on manual (high pressure) for 12 minutes. Allow the natural pressure release for 10 minutes.

Nutritional info per serve: calories 310, fat 17.1, fiber 1.7, carbs 4.4, protein 34.2

Lamb Shank with Spices

Prep time: 15 minutes | **Cook time:** 35 minutes | **Yield:** 2 servings

Ingredients

- 2 lamb shanks
- ¼ teaspoon chili powder
- 1 rosemary spring
- 1 teaspoon coconut flour
- ¼ teaspoon onion powder
- ¾ teaspoon ground ginger
- ½ cup beef broth
- ½ teaspoon avocado oil

Method

1. Put all ingredients in the instant pot.
2. Close and seal the lid.
3. Cook the meat on manual mode (high pressure) for 35 minutes.
4. Then allow the natural pressure release for 15 minutes.

Nutritional info per serve: calories 179, fat 7, fiber 0.8, carbs 2, protein 25.4

Pesto Rack of Lamb

Prep time: 15 minutes | **Cook time:** 45 minutes | **Yield:** 4 servings

Ingredients

- 2 tablespoons pesto sauce
- 1 tablespoon coconut oil
- 1 teaspoon chili powder
- 1-pound rack of lamb
- 1 cup of water

Method

1. Rub the rack of lamb with pesto sauce and chili powder. Leave the meat for 15 minutes to marinate.
2. Then heat up coconut oil on saute mode for 3 minutes.
3. Put the marinated lamb in the hot oil and cook it on saute mode for 4 minutes from each side.
4. Then add water. Close and seal the lid.
5. Cook the lamb on manual (high pressure) for 45 minutes. Make a quick pressure release.

Nutritional info per serve: calories 256, fat 16.8, fiber 0.4, carbs 0.9, protein 23.9

Koobideh

Prep time: 15 minutes | **Cook time:** 30 minutes | **Yield:** 4 servings

Ingredients

- 1-pound ground lamb
- 1 teaspoon ground turmeric
- ½ teaspoon ground black pepper
- 1 tablespoon lemon juice
- 1 teaspoon chives, chopped
- ½ teaspoon garlic powder
- 1 egg, beaten
- 1 cup water, for cooking

Method

1. In the mixing bowl mix up all ingredients from the list above.
2. Then make the meatballs and press them well to get the shape of an ellipse.
3. Then pour water and insert the steamer rack in the instant pot.
4. Put the prepared ellipse meatballs in the baking mold and transfer it on the steamer rack.
5. Close and seal the lid and cook the meal on manual mode (high pressure) for 30 minutes. Make a quick pressure release.

Nutritional info per serve: calories 231, fat 9.5, fiber 0.3, carbs 1, protein 33.4

Shami Kabob

Prep time: 15 minutes | **Cook time:** 40 minutes | **Yield:** 4 servings

Ingredients

- 1-pound beef chunks
- ¼ cup almond flour
- 1 teaspoon ginger paste
- ½ teaspoon ground

- cumin
- 2 cups of water
- 1 tablespoon coconut oil
- 1 egg, beaten

Method

1. Chop the beef chunks and put them in the instant pot.
2. Add ginger paste, ground cumin, and water.
3. Cook the meat on manual mode (high pressure) for 30 minutes. Make a quick pressure release.
4. Drain the water from the meat.
5. Then transfer the beef in the blender. Add almond flour. Blend the ingredients until smooth. Make the small meatballs.
6. Heat up coconut oil on saute mode and put the meatballs inside.
7. Cook them for 2 minutes from each side or until golden brown.

   Nutritional info per serve: calories 179, fat 9.5, fiber 0.3, carbs 2.9, protein 20.1

Lamb Burger

Prep time: 10 minutes | **Cook time:** 14 minutes | **Yield:** 2 servings

Ingredients

- 10 oz ground lamb
- 1 teaspoon garlic powder
- ½ teaspoon chili powder
- 1 teaspoon dried

- cilantro
- ½ teaspoon salt
- ¼ cup of water
- 1 tablespoon coconut oil

Method

1. In the mixing bowl, mix up ground lamb, garlic powder, chili powder, dried cilantro, salt, and water.
2. Make 2 burgers from the lamb mixture.
3. Melt the coconut oil on saute mode.
4. Then put the burgers in the hot oil and cook them for 7 minutes from each side.

   Nutritional info per serve: calories 329, fat 17.3, fiber 0.4, carbs 1.4, protein 40.1

Steamed Rostelle

Prep time: 20 minutes | **Cook time:** 30 minutes | **Yield:** 4 servings

Ingredients

- 1-pound lamb loin
- 1 teaspoon ground black pepper
- 1 teaspoon olive oil

- ½ teaspoon apple cider vinegar
- ½ teaspoon salt
- 1 cup water, for cooking

Method

1. Slice the lamb loin into the medium size strips and sprinkle with ground black pepper, olive oil, apple cider vinegar, and salt.
2. Mix up the meat well.
3. Then sting it on the skewers and put in the baking pan.
4. Pour water in the instant pot and then insert the steamer rack.
5. Put the baking mold with skewers on the rack. Close and seal the lid.
6. Cook the meal on manual (high pressure) for 30 minutes. Allow the natural pressure release for 10 minutes.

   Nutritional info per serve: calories 241, fat 12.3, fiber 0.1, carbs 0.4, protein 30.2

Peppered Lamb Ribs

Prep time: 20 minutes | **Cook time:** 35 minutes | **Yield:** 4 servings

Ingredients

- 1-pound lamb ribs, chopped
- 1 teaspoon peppercorn, grinded
- ¼ cup apple cider vinegar

- 2 tablespoons coconut aminos
- 1 teaspoon cumin seeds
- 1 cup of water

Method

1. Put all ingredients in the instant pot.
2. Close and seal the lid.
3. Cook the meat on manual mode (high pressure) for 35 minutes.
4. Then allow the natural pressure release for 15 minutes.
5. Serve the lamb ribs with hot gravy from the instant pot.

   Nutritional info per serve: calories 205, fat 10.2, fiber 0.2, carbs 2.2, protein 23.2

Classic Taco Meat

Prep time: 7 minutes | **Cook time:** 15 minutes | **Yield:** 4 servings

Ingredients

- 1 oz scallions, chopped
- 1 ½ cup ground beef
- 1 teaspoon taco seasonings
- 1 tablespoon coconut oil

Method

1. Melt the coconut oil on saute mode.
2. When the oil is hot, add ground beef and saute it for 5 minutes. Stir the meat occasionally.
3. Then sprinkle the meat with taco seasonings and mix up well.
4. Cook the taco meat for 5 minutes more.
5. Add scallions and stir the mixture well. Cook it on saute mode for 5 minutes.

Nutritional info per serve: calories 131, fat 9.5, fiber 0.2, carbs 1, protein 9.9

Ropa Vieja

Prep time: 10 minutes | **Cook time:** 30 minutes | **Yield:** 6 servings

Ingredients

- 1-pound beef chuck roast, chopped
- 1 tablespoon coconut oil
- 1 teaspoon garlic, diced
- 1 teaspoon ground coriander
- 1 teaspoon chili powder
- 1 teaspoon ground paprika
- 1 cup of water
- 1 bell pepper, sliced

Method

1. Pour water in the instant pot.
2. Add beef. Close and seal the lid.
3. Cook the meat on manual mode (high pressure) for 20 minutes.
4. Make a quick pressure release and transfer the meat in the bowl. Clean the instant pot.
5. Shred the meat well and return back in the instant pot.
6. Add coconut oil, garlic, ground coriander, chili powder, and ground paprika.
7. Add sliced bell pepper and mix up the ingredients.
8. Saute the meal for 10 minutes. Stir it with the help of the spatula from time to time.

Nutritional info per serve: calories 303, fat 23.5, fiber 0.6, carbs 2.1, protein 20.1

Veal Meatloaf

Prep time: 20 minutes | **Cook time:** 25 minutes | **Yield:** 4 servings

Ingredients

- 1-pound veal, minced
- 1 tablespoon mustard
- 2 eggs, beaten
- ¼ cup coconut flour
- 1 teaspoon salt
- 1 teaspoon ground cumin
- 1 teaspoon olive oil
- 1 cup water, for cooking

Method

1. In the mixing bowl, mix up minced veal, mustard, eggs, coconut flour, salt, and ground cumin.
2. Then brush the baking mold with olive oil.
3. Put the ground veal mixture in the mold and press it gently to get the shape of a loaf.
4. Then pour water and insert the steamer rack in the instant pot.
5. Put the mold with meatloaf on the rack. Close and seal the lid.
6. Cook the meatloaf on manual mode (high pressure) for 25 minutes. Allow the natural pressure release for 15 minutes.

Nutritional info per serve: calories 281, fat 13.6, fiber 3.5, carbs 6.4, protein 32.2

Beef Bone Broth

Prep time: 20 minutes | **Cook time:** 50 minutes | **Yield:** 4 servings

Ingredients

- 1-pound T-bone beef steak, chopped
- 1 teaspoon salt
- 1 teaspoon peppercorns
- 1 bay leaf
- 3 cups of water

Method

1. Put all ingredients in the instant pot. Close and seal the lid.
2. Then set manual mode (high pressure) and cook the mixture for 50 minutes.
3. Allow the natural pressure release for 15 minutes and open the lid.
4. Strain the cooked mixture and shred the meat.
5. The beef broth should be served with shredded beef.

Nutritional info per serve: calories 303, fat 23.1, fiber 0.2, carbs 0.5, protein 22.1

Ground Beef Okra

Prep time: 10 minutes | **Cook time:** 20 minutes | **Yield:** 4 servings

Ingredients

- 1 cup okra, sliced
- 7 oz ground beef
- 1 teaspoon salt
- 1 cup of water
- 1 tablespoon avocado oil
- 1 teaspoon ground black pepper

Method

1. Heat up avocado oil in the instant pot and add ground beef.
2. Sprinkle it with salt and ground black pepper and saute for 10 minutes.
3. After this, add sliced okra and stir the mixture well.
4. Cook the meal on saute mode for 10 minutes.

   Nutritional info per serve: calories 108, fat 3.6, fiber 1.1, carbs 2.4, protein 15.6

Big Mac Salad

Prep time: 10 minutes | **Cook time:** 9 minutes | **Yield:** 2 servings

Ingredients

- 1 cup lettuce, chopped
- 2 oz dill pickles, sliced
- 5 oz ground beef
- 1 oz scallions, chopped
- ¼ cup Monterey Jack cheese, shredded
- 1 tablespoon sesame oil
- 1 tablespoon heavy cream
- 1 teaspoon ground black pepper

Method

1. In the mixing bowl, mix up ground beef and ground black pepper. Make the mini burgers.
2. Pour sesame oil in the instant pot and saute it for 3 minutes.
3. Place the mini hamburgers in the hot oil and cook them for 3 minutes from each side.
4. Meanwhile, in the big salad bowl mix up chopped lettuce, dill pickles, scallions, shredded cheese, and heavy cream. Shake the salad mixture well.
5. Top the salad with cooked mini burgers.

   Nutritional info per serve: calories 284, fat 18.5, fiber 1.2, carbs 3.5, protein 25.7

Sirloin Roast

Prep time: 10 minutes | **Cook time:** 55 minutes | **Yield:** 4 servings

Ingredients

- 1 teaspoon pot roast seasonings
- 16 oz beef sirloin, roughly chopped
- 1 cup of water
- 1 tablespoon sesame oil

Method

1. Rub the beef sirloin with pot roast seasonings and sesame oil and wrap in the foil.
2. After this, pour water and insert the steamer rack in the instant pot.
3. Place the wrapped meat on the rack. Close and seal the lid.
4. Cook the sirloin on manual mode (high pressure) for 55 minutes.
5. Then make a quick pressure release and open the lid.
6. Slice the sirloin roast into the servings.

   Nutritional info per serve: calories 245, fat 10.5, fiber 0, carbs 0.5, protein 34.7

Mexican Pot Roast

Prep time: 10 minutes | **Cook time:** 55 minutes | **Yield:** 4 servings

Ingredients

- 1 tablespoon Mexican style seasonings
- 12 oz beef chuck pot roast, sliced
- 1 tablespoon butter
- 1 garlic clove, diced
- 1 cup of water

Method

1. Toss the butter in the instant pot.
2. Add garlic and saute the ingredients for 3 minutes.
3. Meanwhile, rub the beef chuck roast with Mexican style seasonings.
4. Place the meat in the garlic butter and saute for 6 minutes from each side.
5. Then add water. Close and seal the lid.
6. Cook the Mexican pot roast for 40 minutes on manual mode (high pressure). Make a quick pressure release.

   Nutritional info per serve: calories 309, fat 23.1, fiber 0, carbs 0.3, protein 23.4

Beef Tips

Prep time: 10 minutes | **Cook time:** 55 minutes | **Yield:** 4 servings

Ingredients

- 1-pound chopped beef
- 1 cup beef broth
- 1 tablespoon almond flour
- 1 teaspoon ground
- black pepper
- ½ teaspoon cayenne pepper
- 1 teaspoon salt
- ½ cup heavy cream

Method

1. Pour beef broth and heavy cream in the instant pot.
2. Add ground black pepper, cayenne pepper, and salt.
3. Then add chopped beef. Close and seal the lid.
4. Cook the beef tips on manual mode (high pressure) for 40 minutes.
5. When the cooking time is finished, allow the natural pressure release for 10 minutes and then remove the meat from the instant pot
6. Add almond flour in the beef liquid and stir until smooth. Cook it on saute mode for 10 minutes.
7. Serve the beef tips with thick beef gravy.

Nutritional info per serve: calories 314, fat 16.5, fiber 1, carbs 2.6, protein 37.5

Low Carb Barbacoa

Prep time: 10 minutes | **Cook time:** 60 minutes | **Yield:** 2 servings

Ingredients

- 1 tablespoon chipotle peppers in Adobo sauce
- 1 cup chicken broth
- 1 tablespoon lemon
- juice
- 1 teaspoon sesame oil
- 8 oz beef sirloin, chopped

Method

1. Put all ingredients in the instant pot. Close and seal the lid.
2. Cook the meal on manual mode (high pressure) for 60 minutes.
3. Then allow the natural pressure release and open the lid.
4. You can shred the meat with the help of the fork if desired.

Nutritional info per serve: calories 255, fat 10.3, fiber 0.5, carbs 0.9, protein 37.1

Bo Kho

Prep time: 20 minutes | **Cook time:** 38 minutes | **Yield:** 4 servings

Ingredients

- 10 oz beef stew meat, chopped
- 1 teaspoon curry powder
- 1 teaspoon tomato paste
- ½ teaspoon ginger
- paste
- ½ cup of coconut milk
- 1 cup of water
- 1 cup turnip, chopped

Method

1. Sprinkle the beef stew meat cubes with curry powder.
2. Then place the meat in the instant pot and cook it on saute mode for 3 minutes.
3. Stir it well and add tomato paste, ginger paste, coconut milk, water, and turnip.
4. Close and seal the lid.
5. Cook Bo Kho for 35 minutes on manual mode (high pressure). Then allow the natural pressure release for 7 minutes.

Nutritional info per serve: calories 213, fat 11.7, fiber 1.5, carbs 4.5, protein 22.6

Cauli Beef Burger

Prep time: 15 minutes | **Cook time:** 15 minutes | **Yield:** 2 servings

Ingredients

- ½ cup cauliflower, shredded
- 5 oz ground beef
- 1 teaspoon garlic salt
- ¼ teaspoon ground cumin
- 1 tablespoon scallions, diced
- 1 egg, beaten
- 1 tablespoon coconut oil
- ¼ cup hot water

Method

1. In the mixing bowl, mix up shredded cauliflower, ground beef, garlic salt, ground cumin, and diced scallions.
2. When the meat mixture is homogenous, add egg and stir it well.
3. Make the burgers from the cauli-meat mixture.
4. After this, heat up the coconut oil on saute mode.
5. Place the burgers in the hot oil in one layer and cook them for 5 minutes from each side.
6. Then add water and close the lid. Cook the meal on saute mode for 5 minutes more.

Nutritional info per serve: calories 235, fat 13.5, fiber 0.9, carbs 2.9, protein 25.1

Thick Beef Gravy

Prep time: 10 minutes | **Cook time:** 35 minutes | **Yield:** 2 servings

Ingredients

- 3 oz Brussel sprouts
- 1 cup beef broth
- 4 oz pork loin, chopped
- ½ daikon, chopped
- 1 teaspoon salt
- 1 tablespoon coconut flour
- 1 tablespoon butter
- 1 cup of water

Method

1. Put all ingredients in the instant pot.
2. Close and seal the lid and cook the mixture on manual mode (high pressure) for 30 minutes.
3. Then make a quick pressure release and open the lid.
4. Blend the mixture with the help of the immersion blender and saute it for 5 minutes.

   Nutritional info per serve: calories 246, fat 15.1, fiber 3.3, carbs 7.1, protein 20.4

Beef Bake with Chives

Prep time: 15 minutes | **Cook time:** 25 minutes | **Yield:** 3 servings

Ingredients

- 12 oz ground beef
- 1 tablespoon chives, chopped
- 1 tablespoon fresh parsley, chopped
- ½ teaspoon salt
- 1 egg, beaten
- 1 cup Mozzarella, shredded
- 1 cup of water

Method

1. In the mixing bowl, mix up ground beef, chives, parsley, salt, and egg.
2. When the mixture is homogenous, transfer it in the big baking ramekin.
3. Top the surface of the meat with Mozzarella and wrap in the foil.
4. Pour water and insert the steamer rack in the instant pot.
5. Place the ramekin with the beef bake on the rack. Close and seal the lid.
6. Cook the meal on manual mode (high pressure) for 25 minutes.
7. Then allow the natural pressure release for 10 minutes.

   Nutritional info per serve: calories 259, fat 10.2, fiber 0.1, carbs 0.6, protein 39

Beef Stuffed Kale

Prep time: 15 minutes | **Cook time:** 30 minutes | **Yield:** 4 servings

Ingredients

- 4 kale leaves
- 8 oz ground beef
- 1 teaspoon chives
- ¼ teaspoon cayenne pepper
- ½ cup chicken broth
- ¼ cup heavy cream
- 1 tablespoon cream cheese

Method

1. In the mixing bowl, mix up ground beef, chives, and cayenne pepper.
2. Then fill and roll the kale leaves with ground beef mixture.
3. Place the kale rolls in the instant pot.
4. Add heavy cream, cream cheese, and chicken broth. Close and seal the lid.
5. Cook the meal on manual mode (high pressure) for 30 minutes + make a quick pressure release.

   Nutritional info per serve: calories 153, fat 7.4, fiber 0.3, carbs 2.2, protein 18.7

Beef Meatloaf with Chives

Prep time: 10 minutes | **Cook time:** 10 minutes | **Yield:** 4 servings

Ingredients

- 10 oz ground beef
- 1 egg, beaten
- ½ teaspoon salt
- 1 teaspoon smoked paprika
- 3 tablespoons water
- 1 tablespoon chives, chopped
- 1 cup water, for cooking

Method

1. In the mixing bowl, mix up ground beef, egg, salt, smoked paprika, 3 tablespoons of water, and chives.
2. Take the loaf pan and place the meat mixture there.
3. Flatten it well to make the shape of the meatloaf.
4. Pour 1 cup of water in the instant pot.
5. Insert the trivet in the instant pot and place the meatloaf pan on it.
6. Cook the meal on High pressure (QPR) for 10 minutes.

   Nutritional info per serve: calories 149, fat 5.6, fiber 0.2, carbs 0.4, protein 23

Creamy Beef Strips

Prep time: 6 minutes | **Cook time:** 20 minutes | **Yield:** 3 servings

Ingredients

- ½ teaspoon salt
- 14 oz beef brisket, cut into the strips
- ½ cup of water
- ½ cup heavy cream
- ½ teaspoon ground black pepper
- 1 tablespoon avocado oil

Method

1. Preheat the instant pot on the "Saute" mode.
2. When it is displayed "hot" – pour avocado oil inside and heat it up.
3. Add the meat.
4. Sprinkle the meat with the ground black pepper and salt.
5. Saute it for 5 minutes. Stir it once per cooking time.
6. Add water and heavy cream.
7. Seal the lid and set the "manual" mode.
8. Put the timer on 15 minutes (High Pressure).
9. Make a quick pressure release.

   Nutritional info per serve: calories 322, fat 16.2, fiber 0.3, carbs 1.1, protein 40.6

Almond Butter Beef

Prep time: 10 minutes | **Cook time:** 60 minutes | **Yield:** 3 servings

Ingredients

- 10 oz beef chuck roast, chopped
- ½ cup almond butter
- ½ teaspoon cayenne pepper
- ½ teaspoon salt
- 1 teaspoon dried basil
- 1 cup of water

Method

1. Place the almond butter in the instant pot and start to preheat it on the "Saute" mode.
2. Meanwhile, mix up together the cayenne pepper, salt, and dried basil.
3. Sprinkle the beef with the spices and transfer the meat in the melted almond butter.
4. Close the instant pot lid and lock it.
5. Set the "Manual" mode and put a timer on 60 minutes (Low Pressure).

   Nutritional info per serve: calories 360, fat 27.8, fiber 0.4, carbs 0.7, protein 25.3

Chili Beef Sticks

Prep time: 15 minutes | **Cook time:** 10 minutes | **Yield:** 2 servings

Ingredients

- ¼ teaspoon ground coriander
- ½ teaspoon salt
- ½ teaspoon chili
- powder
- 6 oz ground beef
- 1 tablespoon avocado oil

Method

1. In the mixing bowl, mix up ground coriander, salt, chili powder, and ground beef.
2. Then brush the instant pot bowl with avocado oil and heat up on saute mode.
3. Meanwhile, make the small beef sticks.
4. Put them in the instant pot and cook on saute mode for 4 minutes from each side or until the beef sticks are light crunchy.
5. Dry the cooked meat sticks with the help of the paper towel.

   Nutritional info per serve: calories 169, fat 6.3, fiber 0.5, carbs 0.8, protein 26

Cumin Chili

Prep time: 5 minutes | **Cook time:** 15 minutes | **Yield:** 2 servings

Ingredients

- 13 oz ground beef
- 1 tablespoon cumin seeds
- ½ teaspoon salt
- 1 tablespoon tomato paste
- ½ teaspoon garlic powder
- 1 cup of water

Method

1. Preheat the instant pot bowl on the "Saute" mode until it is displayed "Hot".
2. Then place the ground beef there.
3. Sprinkle it with the cumin seeds, garlic powder, and salt.
4. Stir gently and saute for 4 minutes.
5. After this, add tomato paste.
6. Add water and close the lid.
7. Saute the chili for 10 minutes.
8. When the chili is cooked – transfer it directly into the serving bowls.

   Nutritional info per serve: calories 362, fat 12.2, fiber 0.7, carbs 3.4, protein 56.9

Cardamom Stew Meat

Prep time: 10 minutes | **Cook time:** 50 minutes | **Yield:** 2 servings

Ingredients

- 9 oz beef stew meat, chopped
- 1 teaspoon ground cardamom
- ½ teaspoon salt
- 1 cup broccoli, chopped
- 1 cup of water

Method

1. Preheat the instant pot on the "Saute" mode.
2. When the title "Hot" is displayed – add chopped beef stew meat and cook it for 4 minutes (for 2 minutes from each side).
3. Then add the ground cardamom, salt, and broccoli.
4. Add water and close the instant pot lid.
5. Saute the stew for 45 minutes – to get the tender taste.

Nutritional info per serve: calories 256, fat 8.2, fiber 1.5, carbs 3.7, protein 40.1

Chinese Beef

Prep time: 8 minutes | **Cook time:** 13 minutes | **Yield:** 2 servings

Ingredients

- 14 oz beef flank steak, sliced
- 1 tablespoon almond flour
- ½ teaspoon minced ginger
- 1 oz scallions, sliced
- 1 tablespoon coconut oil
- ¾ cup of water

Method

1. Toss the beef strips in the almond flour and shake well.
2. Toss the coconut oil in the instant pot bowl and set the "saute" mode.
3. When the coconut oil is melted – add the beef flank steak slices and cook them for 3 minutes. Stir them from time to time.
4. Add minced ginger.
5. Pour the water over the meat and lock the instant pot lid.
6. Press the "Manual" mode (High pressure) and set the timer for 10 minutes.
7. Make a quick pressure release.
8. Top the cooked beef with sliced scallions.

Nutritional info per serve: calories 513, fat 26.2, fiber 1.9, carbs 4.4, protein 63.5

Easy Taco Stuffing

Prep time: 5 minutes | **Cook time:** 11 minutes | **Yield:** 2 servings

Ingredients

1 teaspoon taco seasoning

9 oz ground beef

¼ cup beef broth

1 teaspoon tomato paste

Method

1. Place the ground beef and taco seasonings in the instant pot bowl.
2. Start to saute the meat. Cook it for 5 minutes.
3. After this, add beef broth and tomato paste.
4. Stir it well.
5. Set the "Manual" mode (High pressure) and cook the meat for 6 minutes more.
6. After this, use the quick pressure release method.

Nutritional info per serve: calories 249, fat 8.1, fiber 0.1, carbs 1.6, protein 39.4

Blackberry Beef

Prep time: 15 minutes | **Cook time:** 30 minutes | **Yield:** 2 servings

Ingredients

- 15 oz beef loin, chopped
- 1 tablespoon blackberries
- 1 cup of water
- ½ teaspoon ground cinnamon
- 1/3 teaspoon ground black pepper
- ½ teaspoon salt
- 1 tablespoon butter

Method

1. Pour water in the instant pot bowl.
2. Add chopped beef loin, blackberries, ground cinnamon, salt, and ground black pepper. Add butter.
3. Close the instant pot lid and set the "Meat" mode.
4. Cook the meat for 30 minutes. Then remove the meat from the instant pot. Blend the remaining blackberry mixture.
5. Pour it over the meat.

Nutritional info per serve: calories 372, fat 21, fiber 0.6, carbs 3.7, protein 39.4

Moroccan Anise Stew

Prep time: 5 minutes | **Cook time:** 50 minutes | **Yield:** 3 servings

Ingredients

- ½ cup of coconut milk
- 1 teaspoon butter
- ½ teaspoon dried rosemary
- ¼ teaspoon salt
- ½ teaspoon ground coriander
- 13 oz lamb shoulder, chopped
- 1 teaspoon ground anise
- ¾ cup of water

Method

1. Slice the mushrooms and place them in the instant pot bowl.
2. Add all remaining ingredients. Close and seal the lid.
3. Set "Manual" mode for 45 minutes.
4. When the time is over – make natural pressure release for 10 minutes.

   Nutritional info per serve: calories 332, fat 19.8, fiber 1, carbs 2.4, protein 35.4

Beef Cakes Stew

Prep time: 15 minutes | **Cook time:** 10 minutes | **Yield:** 2 servings

Ingredients

- 10 oz ground beef
- ½ teaspoon white pepper
- ½ teaspoon ground paprika
- ½ cup of water
- ½ teaspoon turmeric
- 1 zucchini, chopped
- 1 teaspoon butter
- 1 tablespoon scallions, chopped

Method

1. Mix up together the ground beef, white pepper, ground paprika, turmeric and make the small meat cakes.
2. Place the meat cakes in the instant pot bowl.
3. Add butter and cook them on saute mode for 2 minutes from each side.
4. Then add chopped scallions, water, and zucchini.
5. Lock the instant pot lid and set "Manual" mode (High Pressure) for 10 minutes. Then make a quick release.
6. Transfer the cooked stew in the bowls.

   Nutritional info per serve: calories 302, fat 11.1, fiber 1.6, carbs 4.5, protein 44.4

Oregano Beef Sirloin

Prep time: 10 minutes | **Cook time:** 15 minutes | **Yield:** 2 servings

Ingredients

- 1 cup of water
- ¼ cup of coconut milk
- 14 oz beef sirloin, chopped
- 1 teaspoon dried oregano

Method

1. Put all ingredients in the instant pot. Close and seal the lid.
2. Cook the meal on "Manual' mode (High pressure) for 15 minutes.
3. Use the quick pressure release.

   Nutritional info per serve: calories 440, fat 19.6, fiber 1, carbs 2.1, protein 61

Vegetable Lasagna with Meat

Prep time: 15 minutes | **Cook time:** 20 minutes | **Yield:** 2 servings

Ingredients

- 1 large zucchini, grated
- 8 oz ground beef
- 1 tablespoon coconut milk
- 1 oz provolone
- cheese, shredded
- ½ tomato, sliced
- 1 teaspoon butter, softened
- 1 cup water, for cooking

Method

1. Grease the lasagna mold with butter.
2. Put ½ part of zucchini in the mold and flatten it.
3. Then add ground beef, coconut milk, and sliced tomato.
4. Then top the ingredients with remaining zucchini and flatten well.
5. Pour water and insert the lasagna mold in the into the instant pot.
6. Close and seal the lid.
7. Cook the meal on manual (high pressure) for 20 minutes. Then make a quick pressure release.

   Nutritional info per serve: calories 323, fat 14.9, fiber 2.1, carbs 6.7, protein 40.3

Succulent Beef Ribs

Prep time: 10 minutes | **Cook time:** 40 minutes | **Yield:** 2 servings

Ingredients

- 10 oz beef ribs
- ¾ cup of water
- 2 tablespoons coconut oil
- 1 teaspoon dried marjoram
- ½ teaspoon salt
- ½ cup chicken broth

Method

1. Rub the beef ribs with the dried marjoram and salt.
2. Place the beef ribs in the instant pot bowl.
3. Add chicken broth and water.
4. Then add coconut oil.
5. Close the lid and set the "Meat" mode. Cook the ribs for 40 minutes.

   Nutritional info per serve: calories 391, fat 22.8, fiber 0.1, carbs 0.4, protein 44.3

BBQ Pulled Beef

Prep time: 10 minutes | **Cook time:** 40 minutes | **Yield:** 2 servings

Ingredients

- 9 oz beef loin
- 1 cup of water
- ½ cup BBQ sauce (keto-friendly)

Method

1. Put all ingredients in the instant pot.
2. Close and seal the lid.
3. Cook the beef on manual (high pressure) for 40 minutes.
4. Then make a quick pressure release and shred the beef with the help of the forks.

   Nutritional info per serve: calories 267, fat 13.2, fiber 1, carbs 3, protein 35.1

Pork

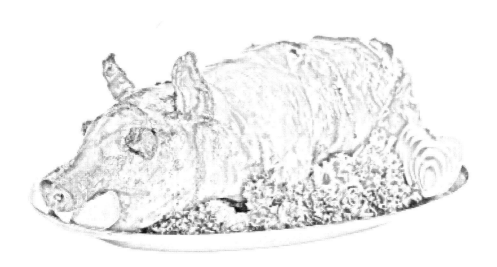

Pork Chops with Blue Cheese

Prep time: 5 minutes | **Cook time:** 20 minutes | **Yield:** 2 servings

Ingredients

- 2 pork chops
- 2 oz blue cheese, crumbled
- 1 teaspoon coconut
- oil
- 1 teaspoon lemon juice
- ¼ cup heavy cream

Method

1. Heat up coconut oil in the instant pot on saute mode.
2. Then put the pork chops in the instant pot and cook them on saute mode for 5 minutes from each side.
3. Then add lemon juice and crumbled cheese.
4. Stir the ingredients well.
5. Add heavy cream and close the lid.
6. Cook the pork chops on saute mode for 10 minutes more.

Nutritional info per serve: calories 300, fat 25.9, fiber 0, carbs 1.1, protein 15.4

Carnitas Pulled Pork

Prep time: 20 minutes | **Cook time:** 45 minutes | **Yield:** 5 servings

Ingredients

- 1-pound pork shoulder, boneless
- ½ teaspoon minced garlic
- ½ teaspoon ground cumin
- 2 tablespoons butter
- 1 chili pepper, chopped
- ½ teaspoon lime zest, grated
- 1 ½ cup beef broth

Method

1. Put all ingredients in the instant pot.
2. Close and seal the lid.
3. Cook the pork for 45 minutes on manual mode (high pressure).
4. Then allow the natural pressure release for 10 minutes and open the lid.
5. Shred the cooked pork with the help of the forks and transfer in the bowl.
6. Add ½ part of all remaining liquid and stir the pulled pork.

Nutritional info per serve: calories 319, fat 24.5, fiber 0.1, carbs 0.6, protein 22.7

Sweet Pork Tenderloin

Prep time: 15 minutes | **Cook time:** 30 minutes | **Yield:** 2 servings

Ingredients

- 9 oz pork tenderloin
- 1 teaspoon Erythritol
- ½ teaspoon dried dill
- ½ teaspoon white
- pepper
- 1 garlic clove, minced
- 3 tablespoons butter
- ¼ cup of water

Method

1. Rub the pork tenderloin with Erythritol, dried dill, white pepper, and minced garlic.
2. Then melt the butter in the instant pot on saute mode.
3. Add pork tenderloin and cook it for 8 minutes from each side (use saute mode).
4. Then add water and close the lid.
5. Cook the meat on saute mode for 10 minutes.
6. Cool the cooked tenderloin for 10-15 minutes and slice.

Nutritional info per serve: calories 339, fat 21.8, fiber 0.2, carbs 3.5, protein 33.8

Thyme Pork Meatballs

Prep time: 15 minutes | **Cook time:** 16 minutes | **Yield:** 8 servings

Ingredients

- 2 cups ground pork
- 1 teaspoon dried thyme
- ½ teaspoon chili flakes
- ½ teaspoon garlic powder
- 1 tablespoon coconut oil
- ¼ teaspoon ground ginger
- 3 tablespoons almond flour
- ¼ cup of water

Method

1. In the mixing bowl, mix up ground pork, dried thyme, chili flakes, garlic powder, ground ginger, and almond flour.
2. Make the meatballs.
3. Melt the coconut oil in the instant pot on saute mode.
4. Arrange the meatballs in the instant pot in one layer and cook them for 3 minutes from each side.
5. Then add water and cook the meatballs for 10 minutes.

Nutritional info per serve: calories 264, fat 19.2, fiber 0.4, carbs 0.8, protein 20.7

Asian Ribs

Prep time: 15 minutes | **Cook time:** 25 minutes | **Yield:** 3 servings

Ingredients

- ¼ teaspoon ground cardamom
- ½ teaspoon minced ginger
- 4 tablespoons apple cider vinegar
- ¼ teaspoon sesame
- seeds
- 10 oz pork ribs, chopped
- ¼ teaspoon chili flakes
- 1 tablespoon avocado oil

Method

1. In the mixing bowl, mix up ground cardamom. Minced ginger, apple cider vinegar, sesame seeds, chili flakes, and avocado oil.

2. Then brush the pork ribs with the cardamom mixture and leave for 10 minutes to marinate.

3. After this, heat up the instant pot on saute mode for 2 minutes.

4. Add the marinated pork ribs and all remaining marinade.

5. Cook the pork ribs on saute mode for 25 minutes. Flip the ribs on another side every 5 minutes.

Nutritional info per serve: calories 271, fat 17.5, fiber 0.3, carbs 0.9, protein 25.2

BBQ Baby Back Ribs

Prep time: 10 minutes | **Cook time:** 30 minutes | **Yield:** 4 servings

Ingredients

- 1-pound pork baby back ribs, chopped
- ¼ cup keto BBQ sauce
- ½ cup of water
- 1 tablespoon sesame seeds

Method

1. Put the chopped ribs, BBQ sauce, and sesame seeds in the instant pot. Add water.

2. Close and seal the lid.

3. Cook the meal on manual mode (high pressure) for 30 minutes.

4. Then allow the natural pressure release for 10 minutes.

Nutritional info per serve: calories 450, fat 34.9, fiber 0.4, carbs 6.2, protein 26.1

Stuffed Pork Rolls

Prep time: 15 minutes | **Cook time:** 21 minutes | **Yield:** 4 servings

Ingredients

- ¼ cup almonds, chopped
- 12 oz pork fillet
- ¼ cup spinach
- 2 oz Parmesan
- 1 tablespoon avocado oil
- 5 tablespoons beef broth

Method

1. Cut the pork fillet on 4 fillets and beat them with the help of the kitchen hammer.

2. Blend the spinach until smooth.

3. After this, grate Parmesan and mix it up with blended spinach and chopped almonds.

4. Sprinkle the spinach mixture over the fillets and roll them in the "envelops".

5. Heat up avocado oil on saute mode.

6. Place the pork rolls in the hot oil and cook them on saute mode for 3 minutes from each side.

7. After this, add water and cook the meal with the closed lid for 15 minutes. Flip the rolls on another side every 5 minutes to avoid burning.

Nutritional info per serve: calories 286, fat 17.4, fiber 0.9, carbs 2.1, protein 29.9

Mississippi Pork

Prep time: 10 minutes | **Cook time:** 6 hours | **Yield:** 7 servings

Ingredients

- 1 tablespoon ranch dressing mix
- 1 ½ pound pork butt roast, chopped
- 1 cup butter
- 1 chili pepper, chopped
- ½ cup of water

Method

1. Put all ingredients in the instant pot.

2. Close the instant pot and cook the meal for 6 hours on low pressure.

3. When the time is over, shred the meat gently and transfer in the serving plate.

Nutritional info per serve: calories 414, fat 38.4, fiber 0, carbs 0.2, protein 17.5

Vietnamese Pork

Prep time: 10 minutes | **Cook time:** 20 minutes | **Yield:** 2 servings

Ingredients

- 6 oz pork tenderloin
- ½ cup of water
- ¼ teaspoon ground clove
- ¼ teaspoon minced ginger
- 1 teaspoon coconut aminos
- 1 teaspoon olive oil

Method

1. Heat up olive oil on saute mode.

2. Then chop the pork tenderloin roughly and add it in the instant pot.

3. Cook the meat for 2 minutes and flip it on another side.

4. After this, add coconut aminos, minced ginger, ground clove, and water.

5. Close and seal the lid and cook the meat on manual (high pressure) for 15 minutes.

6. Allow the natural pressure release for 10 minutes and transfer the meat in the bowls.

   Nutritional info per serve: calories 146, fat 5.4, fiber 0.1, carbs 0.8, protein 22.3

Wrapped Pork Cubes

Prep time: 15 minutes | **Cook time:** 20 minutes | **Yield:** 4 servings

Ingredients

- 6 oz bacon, sliced
- 10 oz pork tenderloin, cubed
- ½ teaspoon white pepper
- 3 tablespoons butter
- ¾ cup chicken stock

Method

1. Melt the butter on saute mode.

2. Meanwhile, wrap the pork tenderloin cubes in the sliced bacon and sprinkle with white pepper.

3. Put the wrapped pork tenderloin in the melted butter and cook them for 3 minutes from each side.

4. Add chicken stock and close the lid.

5. Cook the pork cubes on saute mode for 14 minutes or until meat is tender.

   Nutritional info per serve: calories 410, fat 29, fiber 0.1, carbs 0.9, protein 34.6

Aromatic Pork Belly

Prep time: 10 minutes | **Cook time:** 75 minutes | **Yield:** 4 servings

Ingredients

- 10 oz pork belly
- 1 teaspoon dried rosemary
- ½ teaspoon dried thyme
- ¼ teaspoon ground cinnamon
- 1 teaspoon salt
- 1 cup of water

Method

1. Rub the pork belly with dried rosemary, thyme, ground cinnamon, and salt and transfer in the instant pot bowl.

2. Add water, close and seal the lid.

3. Cook the pork belly on manual mode (high pressure) for 75 minutes.

4. Remove the cooked pork belly from the instant pot and slice it into servings.

   Nutritional info per serve: calories 329, fat 19.1, fiber 0.3, carbs 0.4, protein 32.7

Herbed Pork Tenderloin

Prep time: 15 minutes | **Cook time:** 18 minutes | **Yield:** 4 servings

Ingredients

- ¼ teaspoon ground cumin
- ½ teaspoon ground nutmeg
- ½ teaspoon dried thyme
- ½ teaspoon ground coriander
- 1 tablespoon sesame oil
- 1-pound pork tenderloin
- 2 tablespoons apple cider vinegar
- 1 cup of water

Method

1. In the mixing bowl, mix up ground cumin, ground nutmeg, thyme, ground coriander, and apple cider vinegar.

2. Then rub the meat with the spice mixture.

3. Heat up sesame oil on saute mode for 2 minutes.

4. Put the pork tenderloin in the hot oil and cook it for 5 minutes from each side or until meat is light brown.

5. Add water.

6. Close and seal the lid. Cook the meat on manual mode (high pressure) for 5 minutes.

7. When the time is finished, allow the natural pressure release for 15 minutes.

   Nutritional info per serve: calories 196, fat 7.5, fiber 0.1, carbs 0.4, protein 29.7

Smothered Pork Chops

Prep time: 10 minutes | **Cook time:** 17 minutes | **Yield:** 4 servings

Ingredients

- 4 pork chops
- 1 teaspoon pork seasonings
- ½ teaspoon ground
- black pepper
- ¼ cup heavy cream
- ½ cup chicken broth
- 1 teaspoon olive oil

Method

1. Heat up olive oil on saute mode for 1 minute.

2. Then place the pork chops in the instant pot and cook them for 3 minutes from each side or until they are light brown.

3. Sprinkle the meat with pork seasonings, ground black pepper, chicken broth, and heavy cream.

4. Close and seal the lid.

5. Cook the meal for 10 minutes on manual mode (high pressure).

6. Make a quick pressure release.

   Nutritional info per serve: calories 298, fat 24, fiber 0.1, carbs 0.6, protein 18.8

Paprika Ribs

Prep time: 10 minutes | **Cook time:** 30 minutes | **Yield:** 4 servings

Ingredients

- 1-pound pork ribs
- 1 tablespoon ground paprika
- 1 teaspoon ground turmeric
- 3 tablespoons avocado oil
- 1 teaspoon salt
- ½ cup beef broth

Method

1. Rub the pork ribs with ground paprika, turmeric, salt, and avocado oil.

2. Then pour the beef broth in the instant pot.

3. Arrange the pork ribs in the instant pot. Close and seal the lid.

4. Cook the pork ribs for 30 minutes on manual mode (high pressure).

5. When the time is finished, make a quick pressure release and chop the ribs into servings.

   Nutritional info per serve: calories 335, fat 21.9, fiber 1.2, carbs 2, protein 31.1

Pork Tenders

Prep time: 10 minutes | **Cook time:** 20 minutes | **Yield:** 6 servings

Ingredients

- 1-pound pork tenderloin, sliced
- ½ cup apple cider vinegar
- 1 teaspoon ground nutmeg
- 1 tablespoon butter
- ½ cup of water

Method

1. Mix up the sliced pork tenderloin with ground nutmeg and put it in the instant pot.

2. Add water, butter, and apple cider vinegar.

3. Close and seal the lid and cook the meat on manual mode (high pressure) for 20 minutes.

4. When the time is finished, make a quick pressure release and open the lid.

   Nutritional info per serve: calories 131, fat 4.7, fiber 0.1, carbs 0.4, protein 19.8

Basil Pork Loin

Prep time: 10 minutes | **Cook time:** 17 minutes | **Yield:** 4 servings

Ingredients

- 1-pound pork loin
- 1 teaspoon dried basil
- 1 tablespoon avocado oil
- 1 teaspoon dried
- thyme
- ½ teaspoon salt
- 2 tablespoons apple cider vinegar
- 1 cup water, for cooking

Method

1. In the shallow bowl, mix up dried basil, avocado oil, thyme, salt, and apple cider vinegar.

2. Then rub the pork loin with the spice mixture and leave the meat for 10 minutes to marinate.

3. Wrap the meat in foil and put on the steamer rack.

4. Pour water and transfer the steamer rack with meat in the instant pot.

5. Close and seal the lid. Cook the meat on manual (high pressure) for 20 minutes. Allow the natural pressure release for 5 minutes.

6. Slice the cooked pork loin.

   Nutritional info per serve: calories 281, fat 16.3, fiber 0.2, carbs 0.4, protein 31.1

Ranch Pork Chops

Prep time: 15 minutes | **Cook time:** 15 minutes | **Yield:** 4 servings

Ingredients

- 1 teaspoon ranch seasonings
- 1 tablespoon olive oil
- 4 pork chops
- 1 cup of water

Method

1. Rub the pork chops with ranch seasonings and olive oil.
2. Then place the meat in the instant pot, add water. Close and seal the lid.
3. Cook the pork chops on manual mode (high pressure) for 15 minutes.
4. Naturally release the pressure and transfer the meat on the plates.

   Nutritional info per serve: calories 289, fat 23.4, fiber 0, carbs 0, protein 18

Meatloaf with Eggs

Prep time: 20 minutes | **Cook time:** 25 minutes | **Yield:** 6 servings

Ingredients

- 1 ½ cup ground pork
- 1 teaspoon chives
- 1 teaspoon salt
- ½ teaspoon ground black pepper
- 3 eggs, hard-boiled, peeled
- 2 tablespoons coconut flour
- 1 tablespoon avocado oil
- 1 cup water, for cooking

Method

1. Brush the loaf mold with avocado oil.
2. After this, in the mixing bowl, mix up ground pork, chives, salt, ground black pepper, and coconut flour.
3. Transfer the mixture in the loaf mold and flatten well.
4. Fill it with hard-boiled eggs.
5. Pour water and insert the steamer rack in the instant pot.
6. Put the meatloaf in the instant pot. Close and seal the lid.
7. Cook the meal on manual (high pressure) for 25 minutes. Allow the natural pressure release for 10 minutes.

   Nutritional info per serve: calories 277, fat 19, fiber 1.2, carbs 2.1, protein 23.3

Cilantro Pork Shoulder

Prep time: 10 minutes | **Cook time:** 85 minutes | **Yield:** 4 servings

Ingredients

- 1-pound pork shoulder, boneless
- ¼ cup fresh cilantro, chopped
- 1 cup of water
- 1 teaspoon salt
- 1 teaspoon coconut oil
- ½ teaspoon mustard seeds

Method

1. Pour water in the instant pot.
2. Add pork shoulder, fresh cilantro, salt, coconut oil, and mustard seeds.
3. Close and seal the lid. Cook the meat on high pressure (manual mode) for 85 minutes.
4. Then make a quick pressure release and open the lid.
5. The cooked meat has to be served with the remaining liquid from the instant pot.

   Nutritional info per serve: calories 343, fat 25.5, fiber 0.1, carbs 0.2, protein 26.5

Pork Ragu

Prep time: 10 minutes | **Cook time:** 15 minutes | **Yield:** 3 servings

Ingredients

- 1 bell pepper, sliced
- ½ zucchini, chopped
- 1 daikon, sliced
- 7 oz pork chops, sliced
- 1 teaspoon almond butter
- ½ cup coconut cream
- ½ teaspoon cayenne pepper

Method

1. Melt the almond butter in the instant pot on saute mode.
2. Add sliced pork chops and sprinkle them with cayenne pepper.
3. Cook the meat for 5 minutes.
4. Then flip it on another side and add chopped zucchini and sliced bell pepper.
5. Add daikon and coconut cream.
6. Close and seal the lid.
7. Cook the pork ragu on high pressure (manual mode) for 10 minutes. Make a quick pressure release.

   Nutritional info per serve: calories 359, fat 29.2, fiber 2.7, carbs 8.2, protein 18.1

Apple Cider Vinegar Ham

Prep time: 10 minutes | **Cook time:** 10 minutes | **Yield:** 6 servings

Ingredients

- 1-pound bone-in ham, cooked
- 1 cup apple cider vinegar
- 2 tablespoons Erythritol
- 2 tablespoons butter
- 1 tablespoon avocado oil
- ½ teaspoon pumpkin pie spices

Method

1. Pour apple cider vinegar in the instant pot and insert the steamer rack.

2. Then rub the ham with Erythritol, butter, avocado oil, and pumpkin pie spices.

3. Put the ham on the rack. Close and seal the lid.

4. Cook the ham on high pressure (manual mode) for 10 minutes.

5. Allow the natural pressure release for 5 minutes and open the lid.

6. Slice the ham.

Nutritional info per serve: calories 134, fat 5.4, fiber 0.1, carbs 6.9, protein 16.5

Turmeric Pork Strips

Prep time: 10 minutes | **Cook time:** 22 minutes | **Yield:** 4 servings

Ingredients

- 1-pound pork loin
- 1 teaspoon ground turmeric
- 1 teaspoon coconut
- oil
- ½ teaspoon salt
- ½ cup organic almond milk

Method

1. Cut the pork loin into the strips and sprinkle with salt and ground turmeric.

2. Heat up the coconut oil on saute mode for 1 minute and add pork strips.

3. Saute them for 6 minutes. Stir the meat from time to time.

4. After this, add almond milk and close the lid.

5. Saute the pork for 15 minutes.

Nutritional info per serve: calories 226, fat 11, fiber 0.1, carbs 1.4, protein 30.5

Fabulous Cilantro Meatballs

Prep time: 10 minutes | **Cook time:** 15 minutes | **Yield:** 3 servings

Ingredients

- 1 cup ground pork
- 1 oz fresh cilantro, chopped
- 1 garlic clove, diced
- ½ teaspoon salt
- 1 teaspoon ground coriander
- 2 tablespoons butter
- 1 tablespoon coconut cream

Method

1. Blend the fresh cilantro until it is smooth and mix it up with ground pork, diced garlic, salt, and ground coriander.

2. Make the small meatballs and press them gently with the help of the hand palms.

3. Then melt the butter in the instant pot on saute mode and add the meatballs.

4. Cook them for 3 minutes from each side. Add coconut cream and close the lid.

5. Cook the meal on saute mode for 5 minutes.

Nutritional info per serve: calories 393, fat 30.6, fiber 0.4, carbs 1, protein 27.3

Ground Pork Stroganoff

Prep time: 10 minutes | **Cook time:** 25 minutes | **Yield:** 4 servings

Ingredients

- ½ cup cremini mushrooms, chopped
- 1 teaspoon dried oregano
- ½ teaspoon ground
- nutmeg
- ½ cup of coconut milk
- 1 cup ground pork
- ½ teaspoon salt
- 2 tablespoons butter

Method

1. Heat up butter on saute mode for 3 minutes.

2. Add mushrooms. Saute the vegetables for 5 minutes.

3. Then stir them and add salt, ground pork, ground nutmeg, and dried oregano.

4. Stir the ingredients and cook for 5 minutes more.

5. Add coconut milk and close the lid.

6. Saute the stroganoff for 15 minutes. Stir it from time to time to avoid burning.

Nutritional info per serve: calories 357, fat 29.3, fiber 0.9, carbs 2.4, protein 21.1

Stew Cubes

Prep time: 15 minutes | **Cook time:** 25 minutes | **Yield:** 2 servings

Ingredients

- 10 oz pork tenderloin
- 1 teaspoon tomato paste
- 1 bay leaf
- 1 teaspoon salt
- 1 cup of water
- 1 teaspoon allspices
- 1 teaspoon coconut oil

Method

1. Cut the pork tenderloin into the cubes and sprinkle with salt and allspices.
2. Then heat up the coconut oil in the instant pot on saute mode. Add pork cubes.
3. Roast the meat for 2 minutes per side.
4. Add tomato paste and water.
5. Close and seal the lid.
6. Cook the stew cubes for 25 minutes on manual mode (high pressure).
7. When the cooking time is finished, allow the natural pressure release for 10 minutes.

   Nutritional info per serve: calories 229, fat 7.4, fiber 0.5, carbs 1.6, protein 37.3

Pork Milanese

Prep time: 10 minutes | **Cook time:** 20 minutes | **Yield:** 2 servings

Ingredients

- 2 bone-in pork chops
- 1 teaspoon salt
- 1 teaspoon ground black pepper
- ½ cup coconut flakes
- 1 oz Parmesan, grated
- 2 eggs, beaten
- 1 teaspoon onion powder
- 1/3 cup butter

Method

1. Rub the pork chops with salt and ground black pepper.
2. In the mixing bowl, mix up coconut flakes, onion powder, and grated Parmesan.
3. Then dip the pork chops in the beaten eggs and coat in the coconut flakes mixture.
4. Melt the butter in the instant pot on saute mode.
5. Add the pork chops and cook them for 10 minutes from each side.

   Nutritional info per serve: calories 697, fat 56.8, fiber 2.2, carbs 6.6, protein 40.3

Romano Pork Chops

Prep time: 10 minutes | **Cook time:** 18 minutes | **Yield:** 3 servings

Ingredients

- 3 pork chops
- 4 oz Romano cheese, grated
- ½ teaspoon Cajun seasoning
- 1 egg, beaten
- 1 tablespoon cream cheese
- 1/3 cup almond flour
- 3 tablespoons avocado oil

Method

1. Rub the pork chops with Cajun seasonings.
2. After this, in the mixing bowl mix up grated Romano cheese and almond flour.
3. In the separated bow mix up eggs and cream cheese.
4. Dip the pork chops in the egg mixture and then coat in the cheese mixture.
5. Repeat the step one more time.
6. Pour avocado oil in the instant pot. Preheat it on saute mode for 2 minutes.
7. Add the pork chops and cook them for 8 minutes per side.

   Nutritional info per serve: calories 528, fat 40.4, fiber 1.9, carbs 5, protein 35

Peppercorn Pork

Prep time: 10 minutes | **Cook time:** 12 minutes | **Yield:** 3 servings

Ingredients

- 3 pork chops
- 1 tablespoon mascarpone cheese
- 1 teaspoon peppercorns, grinded
- ½ teaspoon dried sage
- 1 tablespoon sunflower oil

Method

1. In the shallow bowl, mix up peppercorns, dried sage, sunflower oil, and mascarpone cheese.
2. Brush the pork chops with the cheese mixture well and transfer in the instant pot.
3. Cook the meat on saute mode for 5 minutes from each side.
4. Then add the remaining cream cheese mixture and cook the pork chops for 2 minutes more.

   Nutritional info per serve: calories 308, fat 25.3, fiber 0.2, carbs 0.7, protein 18.7

Ground Pork Pizza Crust

Prep time: 10 minutes | **Cook time:** 15 minutes | **Yield:** 4 servings

Ingredients

- ½ cup Cheddar cheese, shredded
- 1 cup ground pork
- 1 teaspoon Italian seasonings
- 1 tablespoon Psyllium husk
- 1 teaspoon olive oil
- 1 cup water, for cooking

Method

1. In the mixing bowl, mix up shredded cheese, ground pork, Italian seasonings, and Psyllium husk.
2. Line the round instant pot pan with baking paper and brush with olive oil.
3. Then put the ground pork mixture in the pan and flatten it in the shape of the pizza crust.
4. Pour water and insert the steamer rack in the instant pot.
5. Put the pan with pizza crust on the rack. Close and seal the lid.
6. Cook the meal on manual mode (high pressure) for 15 minutes. Make a quick pressure release.

Nutritional info per serve: calories 324, fat 22.5, fiber 7, carbs 8.8, protein 23.6

Pork Chops Al Pastor

Prep time: 10 minutes | **Cook time:** 30 minutes | **Yield:** 4 servings

Ingredients

- 4 pork chops
- 1 teaspoon Achiote paste
- 1 teaspoon minced garlic
- 1 tablespoon avocado oil
- 2 tablespoon lime juice
- ½ cup chicken broth

Method

1. In the shallow bowl, mix up Achiote paste, minced garlic, avocado oil, and lime juice.
2. Then rub the pork chops with the Achiote paste mixture and put in the instant pot.
3. Cook the meat on Saute mode for 6 minutes from each side.
4. Add chicken broth and close the lid.
5. Cook the meal on Saute mode for 20 minutes.

Nutritional info per serve: calories 279, fat 21.5, fiber 0.2, carbs 1.1, protein 18.9

Taco Casserole

Prep time: 20 minutes | **Cook time:** 30 minutes | **Yield:** 4 servings

Ingredients

- 1 cup ground pork
- 1 tablespoon taco seasonings
- 1 tablespoon coconut oil
- ½ teaspoon dried cilantro
- ¼ cup Cheddar cheese, shredded
- ½ cup beef broth

Method

1. In the mixing bowl, mix up ground pork, taco seasonings, and dried cilantro.
2. Then grease the casserole mold with coconut oil and put the pork mixture inside. Flatten it well.
3. After this, top the casserole mixture with shredded cheese.
4. Add beef broth and cover the casserole with foil.
5. Pour water in the instant pot and place the casserole inside.
6. Close and seal the lid.
7. Cook the meal on manual (high pressure) for 30 minutes.
8. Allow the natural pressure release for 10 minutes.

Nutritional info per serve: calories 302, fat 22.2, fiber 0, carbs 1.7, protein 22.5

Pork and Sauerkraut Mix

Prep time: 10 minutes | **Cook time:** 15 minutes | **Yield:** 4 servings

Ingredients

- 4 pork chops, chopped
- ½ teaspoon cayenne pepper
- ½ teaspoon ground coriander
- 1 tablespoon coconut oil
- 1 tablespoon avocado oil
- 1 cup sauerkraut

Method

1. Melt the coconut oil on saute mode.
2. Add cayenne pepper, ground coriander, and chopped pork chops.
3. Cook the meat on saute mode for 7 minutes from each side.
4. Then transfer the cooked meat in the bowl, add sauerkraut and mix up well.

Nutritional info per serve: calories 297, fat 23.8, fiber 1.2, carbs 1.9, protein 18.4

Mozzarella Stuffed Meatballs

Prep time: 10 minutes | **Cook time:** 20 minutes | **Yield:** 6 servings

Ingredients

- 1-pound ground pork
- 1 teaspoon chili flakes
- ½ teaspoon salt
- 1/3 cup Mozzarella, shredded
- 1 tablespoon butter
- ¼ cup chicken broth
- ½ teaspoon garlic powder

Method

1. Mix up ground pork, chili flakes, salt, and garlic powder.
2. Then make the meatballs with the help of the fingertips.
3. Make the mini balls from the cheese.
4. Fill the meatballs with the mini cheese balls.
5. Toss the butter in the instant pot.
6. Heat it up on saute mode and add the prepared meatballs.
7. Cook the on saute mode for 3 minutes from each side.
8. Then add chicken broth and close the lid.
9. Cook the meal on meat/stew mode for 10 minutes.

   Nutritional info per serve: calories 132, fat 4.9, fiber 0, carbs 0.3, protein 20.5

Bacon Sticks

Prep time: 5 minutes | **Cook time:** 5 minutes | **Yield:** 4 servings

Ingredients

- 2 tablespoons almond flour
- 1 tablespoon water
- 6 oz bacon, sliced
- ¾ teaspoon chili pepper

Method

1. Sprinkle the sliced bacon with the almond flour and water. Add chili pepper.
2. Put it in the instant pot in one layer.
3. Cook the meal on the "Saute" program for 6 minutes (cook for 3 minutes per side).

   Nutritional info per serve: calories 251, fat 19.4, fiber 0.4, carbs 1.5, protein 16.5

Smoked Sausages Cabbage

Prep time: 15 minutes | **Cook time:** 20 minutes | **Yield:** 2 servings

Ingredients

- 1 cup white cabbage, shredded
- 6 oz smoked sausages, chopped
- 1 teaspoon avocado oil
- 1 teaspoon ground paprika
- ½ teaspoon chili powder
- 1 cup chicken stock

Method

1. Put the smoked sausages and avocado oil in the instant pot and cook the ingredients on saute mode for 5 minutes. Stir them from time to time.
2. After this, add ground paprika, chili powder, and shredded cabbage. Mix up well.
3. Add chicken stock. Close and seal the lid.
4. Cook the meal on manual mode (high pressure) for 15 minutes.
5. Then make a quick pressure release.
6. Stir the meal well before serving.

   Nutritional info per serve: calories 310, fat 25, fiber 1.6, carbs 3.5, protein 17.6

Sub Salad

Prep time: 10 minutes | **Cook time:** 15 minutes | **Yield:** 4 servings

Ingredients

- 1 tomato, chopped
- 1/3 cup black olives, sliced
- 1 cup lettuce, chopped
- 1 tablespoon olive oil
- ½ teaspoon chicken seasonings
- 10 oz pork fillet
- 1/3 cup water, for cooking

Method

1. Slice the pork fillet and sprinkle with chicken seasonings.
2. Then place the sliced meat in the instant pot, add olive oil and cook on saute mode for 5 minutes.
3. Stir it from time to time.
4. When the meat is light brown, add water and close the lid.
5. Cook it on meat/stew mode for 10 minutes.
6. Meanwhile, in the salad bowl, mix up tomato, black olives, and lettuce.
7. Top the salad with the cooked pork slices.

   Nutritional info per serve: calories 213, fat 13.8, fiber 0.6, carbs 1.7, protein 20

Pork Chops Marsala

Prep time: 20 minutes | **Cook time:** 25 minutes |
Yield: 2 servings

Ingredients

- 2 pork chops
- ½ cup cremini mushrooms, sliced
- ¼ cup apple cider vinegar
- 1 tablespoon coconut oil
- 1 teaspoon dried thyme
- ½ cup heavy cream
- ¼ cup chicken broth

Method

1. Put all ingredients in the instant pot.
2. Close and seal the lid.
3. Cook the pork on manual mode (high pressure) for 25 minutes.
4. Allow the natural pressure release for 15 minutes and open the lid.
5. Stir the pork chop marsala well before serving.

Nutritional info per serve: calories 435, fat 38, fiber 0.3, carbs 2.3, protein 19.7

Pork Florentine

Prep time: 20 minutes | **Cook time:** 45 minutes |
Yield: 6 servings

Ingredients

- 12 oz pork roast, roll cut
- 1 cup spinach
- 3 oz Monterey Jack cheese, shredded
- 1 tablespoon olive oil
- ½ teaspoon ground black pepper
- 1 cup water, for cooking

Method

1. Beet the pork roast with the help of the kitchen hammer.
2. After this, put the spinach in the blender and add olive oil, and ground black pepper. Blend the mixture until smooth.
3. Then transfer the mixture over the pork roast, spread it well and top with shredded cheese.
4. Roll the meat and wrap in the foil.
5. Pour water and insert the steamer rack in the instant pot.
6. Put the wrapped pork on the steamer rack. Close and seal the lid.
7. Cook the meal on manual mode (high pressure) for 45 minutes.
8. Allow the natural pressure release for 15 minutes.

Nutritional info per serve: calories 298, fat 20.6, fiber 0.2, carbs 0.6, protein 26.7

Ground Salisbury Steak

Prep time: 10 minutes | **Cook time:** 25 minutes |
Yield: 4 servings

Ingredients

- 1 cup ground pork
- 1 teaspoon chili flakes
- 1 teaspoon dried cilantro
- 1 cup chicken broth
- 1 teaspoon olive oil
- 1 tablespoon mustard
- 1 cup white mushrooms, chopped

Method

1. Put olive oil and mushrooms in the instant pot.
2. Add dried cilantro, and chili flakes and cook the ingredients for 10 minutes on saute mode.
3. Then add mustard and ground pork.
4. Add chicken broth. Close and seal the lid.
5. Cook the meat on manual mode (high pressure) for 15 minutes.
6. Make a quick pressure release.

Nutritional info per serve: calories 94, fat 6.4, fiber 0.6, carbs 1.8, protein 7.5

Garlic Italian Sausages

Prep time: 15 minutes | **Cook time:** 20 minutes |
Yield: 4 servings

Ingredients

- 1 teaspoon garlic powder
- 1 cup of water
- 1 teaspoon butter
- 12 oz Italian sausages, chopped
- ½ teaspoon Italian seasonings

Method

1. Sprinkle the chopped Italian sausages with Italian seasonings and garlic powder and place in the instant pot.
2. Add butter and cook the sausages on saute mode for 10 minutes. Stir them from time to time with the help of the spatula.
3. Then add water and close the lid.
4. Cook the sausages on manual mode (high pressure) for 10 minutes.
5. Allow the natural pressure release for 10 minutes more.

Nutritional info per serve: calories 307, fat 27.8, fiber 0.1, carbs 1.1, protein 12.3

Adobo Pork

Prep time: 10 minutes | **Cook time:** 30 minutes | **Yield:** 6 servings

Ingredients

- 1-pound pork belly, chopped
- 1 bay leaf
- 1 teaspoon salt
- 2 tablespoons apple cider vinegar
- 1 teaspoon cayenne pepper
- 1 garlic clove, peeled
- 2 cups of water

Method

1. Put all ingredients in the instant pot.
2. Close and seal the lid.
3. Cook Adobo pork for 30 minutes on manual mode (high pressure).
4. When the cooking time is finished, make a quick pressure release and transfer the pork belly in the bowls.
5. Add 1 ladle of the pork gravy.

Nutritional info per serve: calories 352, fat 20.4, fiber 0.1, carbs 0.5, protein 35

Cuban Pork

Prep time: 20 minutes | **Cook time:** 35 minutes | **Yield:** 3 servings

Ingredients

- 9 oz pork shoulder, boneless, chopped
- 1 tablespoon avocado oil
- 1 teaspoon ground cumin
- ½ teaspoon ground black pepper
- ¼ cup apple cider vinegar
- 1 cup of water

Method

1. In the mixing bowl, mix up avocado oil, ground cumin, ground black pepper, and apple cider vinegar.
2. Mix up pork shoulder and spice mixture together and transfer on the foil. Wrap the meat mixture.
3. Pour water and insert the steamer rack in the instant pot.
4. Put the wrapped pork shoulder on the rack. Close and seal the lid.
5. Cook the Cuban pork for 35 minutes.
6. Then allow the natural pressure release for 10 minutes.

Nutritional info per serve: calories 262, fat 19, fiber 0.4, carbs 1, protein 20

Kalua Pork

Prep time: 10 minutes | **Cook time:** 10 hours | **Yield:** 4 servings

Ingredients

- 1-pound pork butt
- 1 teaspoon salt
- ½ teaspoon liquid smoke
- 1 cucumber, chopped
- 1 tomato, chopped
- ½ bell pepper, chopped

Method

1. Rub the meat with salt and liquid smoke and put it in the instant pot.
2. Close the lid and cook it on "low" for 10 hours.
3. Meanwhile, mix up together cucumber, tomato, and bell pepper.
4. Shred the cooked meat and put it in the serving bowls.
5. Top the meat with vegetable mixture.

Nutritional info per serve: calories 238, fat 7.7, fiber 0.8, carbs 4.5, protein 36.1

Pork Loin in Vegetable Gravy

Prep time: 10 minutes | **Cook time:** 50 minutes | **Yield:** 4 servings

Ingredients

1-pound pork loin

- ½ cup cauliflower, chopped
- 1 daikon, chopped
- 2 oz celery stalk, chopped
- 1 teaspoon salt
- 1 teaspoon peppercorns
- 2 cups of water
- 1 tablespoon almond flour

Method

1. Put the pork loin in the instant pot.
2. Add cauliflower, chopped daikon, celery stalk, salt, peppercorns, and water.
3. Close and seal the lid and cook the meat on manual mode (high pressure) for 40 minutes.
4. Then make a quick pressure release and open the lid.
5. Transfer the meat on the plate.
6. Add the almond flour in the remaining mixture in the instant pot and with the help of the immersion blender, blend the mixture until smooth.
7. Saute the gravy for 10 minutes.
8. Pour the cooked gravy over the meat.

Nutritional info per serve: calories 324, fat 19.3, fiber 1.7, carbs 3.4, protein 33.1

Light Posole

Prep time: 10 minutes | **Cook time:** 35 minutes | **Yield:** 4 servings

Ingredients

- 1 teaspoon Ancho chili powder
- ½ teaspoon ground coriander
- ½ teaspoon of cocoa powder
- 1-pound pork shoulder, boneless, chopped
- 2 cups beef broth

Method

1. Put ground coriander, beef broth, and cocoa powder in the instant pot.
2. Stir the mixture until the beef broth will turn color into chocolate.
3. Add Ancho chili powder, and pork shoulder.
4. Close the lid.
5. Cook the meal on meat/stew mode for 35 minutes.

Nutritional info per serve: calories 351, fat 25, fiber 0.1, carbs 0.6, protein 28.9

Sweet Ham

Prep time: 10 minutes | **Cook time:** 7 minutes | **Yield:** 6 servings

Ingredients

- 1-pound ham
- ½ cup butter
- 3 tablespoons Erythritol
- ½ teaspoon cumin seeds
- 1 cup water, for cooking

Method

1. Pour water in the instant pot and insert the steamer rack.
2. After this, in the mixing bowl, mix up Erythritol, butter, and cumin seeds.
3. Brush the ham with the sweet mixture well and transfer it in the instant pot.
4. Add the remaining sweet mixture. Close and seal the lid.
5. Cook the ham on manual mode (high pressure) for 7 minutes.
6. Make a quick pressure release and slice the ham.

Nutritional info per serve: calories 260, fat 21.9, fiber 1, carbs 3, protein 12.7

Tangy Pork

Prep time: 10 minutes | **Cook time:** 40 minutes | **Yield:** 3 servings

Ingredients

- 8 oz pork loin
- 1 teaspoon keto ketchup
- 1 cup of water
- 3 tablespoons coconut aminos
- ½ teaspoon garlic powder
- 1 tablespoon Splenda
- ½ teaspoon cayenne pepper

Method

1. Cut the pork loin on 3 servings and put in the instant pot.
2. Add keto ketchup, water, coconut aminos, garlic powder, Splenda, and cayenne pepper.
3. Stir the mixture gently and close the lid.
4. Cook the tangy pork on meat/stew mode for 40 minutes.

Nutritional info per serve: calories 222, fat 10.6, fiber 0.1, carbs 7.9, protein 20.8

Pork Dumpling Meatballs

Prep time: 10 minutes | **Cook time:** 19 minutes | **Yield:** 2 servings

Ingredients

- 6 oz ground pork
- 1 teaspoon minced garlic
- ½ teaspoon chives, chopped
- 1 teaspoon coconut aminos
- ½ teaspoon cayenne pepper
- 1 tablespoon coconut oil
- 1 teaspoon ginger paste
- ½ cup chicken broth

Method

1. In the bowl, mix up ground pork, minced garlic, chives, coconut aminos, cayenne pepper, and ginger paste.
2. Make the small balls (dumplings) from the meat mixture.
3. After this, melt the coconut oil and put the meatballs inside.
4. Roast them on saute mode for 1 minute from each side.
5. Then add chicken broth and close the lid.
6. Saute the meal on saute mode for 15 minutes.

Nutritional info per serve: calories 199, fat 10.3, fiber 0.3, carbs 2.1, protein 23.7

Tender Pork Liver

Prep time: 5 minutes | **Cook time:** 7 minutes | **Yield:** 3 servings

Ingredients

- 14 oz pork liver, chopped
- ½ cup heavy cream
- 3 tablespoons scallions, chopped
- 1 teaspoon salt
- 1 teaspoon butter

Method

1. Sprinkle the liver with the salt.
2. Toss the butter in the instant pot and melt it on the "Saute" mode.
3. Add heavy cream, scallions, and liver.
4. Stir gently and close the lid.
5. Cook the meal on the "Saute" mode for 12 minutes.

   Nutritional info per serve: calories 300, fat 14.5, fiber 0.2, carbs 6, protein 35

Cheesesteak Meatloaf

Prep time: 15 minutes | **Cook time:** 40 minutes | **Yield:** 4 servings

Ingredients

- 1 cup ground pork
- ½ cup Cheddar cheese, shredded
- 2 tablespoons almond flour
- 1 tablespoon chives, chopped
- 1 teaspoon pork seasonings
- 1 egg, beaten
- 1 cup water, for cooking

Method

1. Put the ground pork in the bowl.
2. Add almond flour, chives, pork seasonings, and egg.
3. Mix up the mixture until smooth.
4. After this, place ½ part of the mixture in the loaf mold, flatten it well and top with ½ part of all Cheddar cheese.
5. Then add remaining ground pork mixture and cheese.
6. Pour water and insert the steamer rack in the instant pot.
7. Place the meatloaf on the rack. Close and seal the lid.
8. Cook the meal on manual mode (high pressure) for 40 minutes. Make a quick pressure release.

   Nutritional info per serve: calories 326, fat 23.7, fiber 0.4, carbs 1, protein 25.8

Eggplant Lasagna

Prep time: 20 minutes | **Cook time:** 30 minutes | **Yield:** 6 servings

Ingredients

- 10 oz ground pork
- 1 cup Mozzarella, shredded
- 1 tablespoon tomato paste
- 2 eggplants, sliced
- 1 teaspoon salt
- 1 teaspoon butter, softened
- 1 cup chicken stock

Method

1. Sprinkle the eggplants with salt and leave for 10 minutes.
2. Then make the eggplants dry with the help of the pepper towel.
3. In the mixing bowl, mix up ground pork, butter, and tomato paste.
4. Make the layer of the sliced eggplants in the instant pot and top it with the thin layer of ground pork mixture.
5. Then top the ground pork with Mozzarella and repeat all the steps again till you use all ingredients.
6. Add chicken stock.
7. Close and seal the lid.
8. Cook the lasagna on manual mode for 30 minutes.
9. Then allow the natural pressure release for 10 minutes and open the lid. Cool the meal for 10 minutes.

   Nutritional info per serve: calories 136, fat 3.6, fiber 6.6, carbs 11.5, protein 15.7

Herbed Butter Pork Chops

Prep time: 5 minutes | **Cook time:** 12 minutes | **Yield:** 5 servings

Ingredients

- 13 oz pork chops
- 1/2 cup butter, softened
- 1 tablespoon Italian seasonings

Method

1. Whisk together Italian seasonings and butter.
2. Rub the pork chops with herbed butter and put in the instant pot.
3. Cook the meat on saute mode for 7 minutes from each side.

   Nutritional info per serve: calories 407, fat 37.6, fiber 0, carbs 0.3, protein 16.8

Filipino Pork

Prep time: 10 minutes | **Cook time:** 40 minutes | **Yield:** 4 servings

Ingredients

- 1-pound pork loin, chopped
- ½ cup apple cider vinegar
- 1 cup chicken broth
- 1 chili pepper, chopped
- 1 tablespoon coconut oil
- 1 teaspoon salt

Method

1. Melt the coconut oil on saute mode.
2. When it is hot, and chili pepper and cook it for 2 minutes. Stir it.
3. Add chopped pork loin and salt. Cook the ingredients for 5 minutes.
4. After this, add apple cider vinegar and chicken broth.
5. Close and seal the lid and cook the Filipino pork for 30 minutes on High pressure (manual mode). Then make a quick pressure release.

Nutritional info per serve: calories 320, fat 19.5, fiber 0, carbs 0.6, protein 32.2

Pork Cubes in Sauce

Prep time: 8 minutes | **Cook time:** 30 minutes | **Yield:** 2 servings

Ingredients

- 1 teaspoon lemon juice
- 10 oz pork loin, chopped
- ½ cup of water
- 1 oz fennel, chopped
- 1 teaspoon salt
- ½ teaspoon peppercorns

Method

1. Sprinkle the chopped pork loin with the lemon juice.
2. Then strew the meat with the salt.
3. Place the meat in the meat mold.
4. Insert the meat mold in the instant pot.
5. Add water, fennel, and peppercorns.
6. Close the lid and lock it.
7. Set the "Meat" mode and put a timer on 30 minutes.
8. Serve the pork cubes with hot gravy.

Nutritional info per serve: calories 349, fat 19.8, fiber 0.6, carbs 1.4, protein 39

Pork Eggplant Halves

Prep time: 15 minutes | **Cook time:** 5 minutes | **Yield:** 2 servings

Ingredients

- 1 eggplant, halved
- 10 oz ground pork
- ½ teaspoon minced garlic
- ½ teaspoon salt
- 1 tablespoon butter
- 1 teaspoon tomato paste

Method

1. Remove ½ of pulp from the eggplants.
2. Mix up together the minced garlic, salt, tomato paste, and ground pork.
3. Fill the eggplants with the pork mixture.
4. Cover the eggplant halves with the butter.
5. Wrap the eggplants into the foil and transfer them on the steamer rack in the instant pot.
6. Pour 1 cup of water in the instant pot and close the lid.
7. Cook the eggplants on High Pressure (Steam mode) for 7 minutes.
8. Then make the natural pressure release for 5 minutes.

Nutritional info per serve: calories 314, fat 11.2, fiber 8.2, carbs 14.2, protein 39.6

Ginger Meatballs

Prep time: 10 minutes | **Cook time:** 7 minutes | **Yield:** 2 servings

Ingredients

- 1 teaspoon ginger paste
- 11 oz ground pork
- 1 teaspoon lemon juice
- ¼ teaspoon chili flakes
- 1 tablespoon butter
- ¼ cup of water

Method

1. Combine together the ground pork and ginger paste.
2. Add lemon juice, and chili flakes.
3. Toss the butter in the instant pot bowl and melt it.
4. Meanwhile, make the small meatballs from the meat mixture.
5. Place the meatballs in the instant pot and cook for 2 minutes from each side.
6. After this, add water and lock the lid.
7. Set the "Manual" mode for 3 minutes (High pressure) + Quick pressure release.

Nutritional info per serve: calories 278, fat 11.3, fiber 0.1, carbs 0.7, protein 41

Smoked Paprika Pulled Pork

Prep time: 7 minutes | **Cook time:** 40 minutes | **Yield:** 3 servings

Ingredients

- 1-pound pork roast, chopped
- ½ teaspoon ground cumin
- 1 tablespoon smoked paprika
- 1 cup beef broth
- 1 tablespoon coconut oil
- 1 teaspoon garlic powder

Method

1. Mix up together garlic powder and ground cumin.
2. Then combine together the spices and chopped pork roast. Add the smoked paprika.
3. Place the meat in the instant pot bowl. Add coconut oil and beef broth.
4. Close the instant pot lid and seal it.
5. Set the manual mode and put the timer on 30 minutes (High pressure).
6. Make the natural-release pressure.
7. Transfer the cooked meat in the bowl and shred it. Serve the meal with meat liquid.

Nutritional info per serve: calories 376, fat 19.6, fiber 1, carbs 2.4, protein 45.3

Bell Peppers with Pork

Prep time: 10minutes | **Cook time:** 15 minutes | **Yield:** 2 servings

Ingredients

- 8 oz bell peppers, deseeded
- 5 oz ground beef
- ¼ teaspoon salt
- ¾ teaspoon ground black pepper
- 2 teaspoon cream cheese
- ½ cup of water

Method

1. Mix up together the salt, and ground black pepper. Stir it well.
2. Fill the peppers with the ground beef mixture.
3. Top every pepper with the cream cheese.
4. Pour water in the instant pot and add the steam rack.
5. Place the peppers on the steam rack and close the instant pot lid and seal it.
6. Set the "Manual" mode and put the timer on 9 minutes. Make NPR (appx. 5 minutes).

Nutritional info per serve: calories 169, fat 5.8, fiber 2.2, carbs 6.1, protein 22.9

Chili Pork Cubes

Prep time: 10 minutes | **Cook time:** 20 minutes | **Yield:** 2 servings

Ingredients

- 10 oz pork loin
- ¼ cup of water
- 1 teaspoon chili paste
- ½ teaspoon ground black pepper
- ½ teaspoon salt

Method

1. Chop the pork loin into the medium pieces.
2. Sprinkle the meat with the salt and ground black pepper.
3. add chili paste in the meat.
4. Mix up the meat mixture with the help of the hands.
5. Pour water in the instant pot bowl and add meat mixture.
6. Close the lid and set the "Meat/Stew" mode. Cook the meal for 25 minutes.
7. Then chill the meat until warm.

Nutritional info per serve: calories 353, fat 20.2, fiber 0.1, carbs 1.3, protein 39

Pork Muffins

Prep time: 5 minutes | **Cook time:** 9 minutes | **Yield:** 2 servings

Ingredients

- 2 tablespoons coconut flour
- 1 egg, beaten
- 4 oz ground pork, fried
- 1 teaspoon parsley
- ¼ teaspoon salt
- 1 tablespoon coconut cream

Method

1. Whisk the beaten egg with the help of the hand whisker.
2. Stir the coconut flour into the whisked egg and add parsley, salt, and coconut cream. Add cooked ground pork.
3. Mix up the mixture until homogenous.
4. Pour the mixture into the muffin molds.
5. Pour 1 cup of water in the instant pot and place trivet.
6. Transfer the muffin molds on the trivet and close the instant pot lid.
7. Set the "manual" mode and cook the muffins for 4 minutes of +natural pressure release for 5 minutes.

Nutritional info per serve: calories 160, fat 6.7, fiber 3.2, carbs 5.6, protein 18.8

Egg Balls

Prep time: 5 minutes | **Cook time:** 5 minutes | **Yield:** 3 servings

Ingredients

- 2 eggs
- 4 oz fried bacon, chopped
- 1 tablespoon butter
- ¾ teaspoon salt
- 1 tablespoon cream cheese

Method

1. Pour 1 cup of water in the instant pot bowl and add eggs. Seal the instant pot lid.
2. Set the "Steam" program and cook the eggs for 5 minutes. Then make a quick release.
3. Meanwhile, melt the butter and mix it up with the salt, bacon, and cream cheese.
4. Chill the cooked eggs, peel them, and chop.
5. Stir together eggs and bacon mixture.
6. Make the egg balls.

   Nutritional info per serve: calories 292, fat 23.7, fiber 0, carbs 0.9, protein 18

Pork Quiche

Prep time: 10 minutes | **Cook time:** 6 minutes | **Yield:** 2 servings

Ingredients

- 3 eggs, beaten
- 1 tablespoon coconut flour
- 4 oz Mozzarella, shredded
- 5 oz ground pork
- ¼ cup spinach
- ½ teaspoon salt
- 1 tablespoon butter

Method

1. Whisk the eggs and coconut flour together.
2. add ground pork in the egg mixture.
3. After this, chop the spinach and add in the egg mixture too.
4. Add butter and mix up the mixture very carefully.
5. Place the mixture into the quiche pan. Sprinkle the mixture with Mozzarella over.
6. Then transfer the pan in the instant pot and close the lid.
7. Set the "Manual" program and cook quiche for 6 minutes + QPR.
8. Cut the quiche into halves.

   Nutritional info per serve: calories 422, fat 25.5, fiber 1.6, carbs 5.2, protein 43.5

Spanish Style Pork Shoulder

Prep time: 10 minutes | **Cook time:** 40 minutes | **Yield:** 3 servings

Ingredients

- 12 oz pork shoulder
- ½ cup chili Verde
- 1 tablespoon butter
- ¼ cup beef broth
- ¾ teaspoon ground black pepper
- ½ teaspoon salt

Method

1. Chop the pork shoulder and sprinkle the meat with the ground black pepper and salt.
2. Toss the butter in the instant pot and saute it for 1 minute or until it is melted.
3. After this, add pork shoulder and saute it for 10 minutes.
4. After this, add beef broth and chili Verde.
5. Lock the instant pot lid and seal it.
6. Set the "Bean/Chili" mode and set the timer on 30 minutes (High Pressure).
7. When the time is over – make a natural pressure release.

   Nutritional info per serve: calories 370, fat 28.2, fiber 0.1, carbs 0.4, protein 26.9

Tender Pork with Salsa Verde

Prep time: 10 minutes | **Cook time:** 40 minutes | **Yield:** 3 servings

Ingredients

- 12 oz pork shoulder, sliced
- ½ cup salsa verde
- ½ cup of water
- ¾ teaspoon peppercorns
- ½ teaspoon salt

Method

1. Toss the butter in the instant pot and saute it for 1 minute or until it is melted.
2. After this, add pork shoulder, salt, and peppercorns; saute the ingredients for 10 minutes.
3. After this, add water and salsa verde.
4. Set the "Bean/Chili" mode and set the timer on 30 minutes (High Pressure).
5. When the time is over – make a natural pressure release.

   Nutritional info per serve: calories 342, fat 24.4, fiber 0.3, carbs 2.1, protein 27

Shredded Pork Stew

Prep time: 15 minutes | **Cook time:** 35 minutes | **Yield:** 2 servings

Ingredients

- 16 oz pork chuck roast
- ½ teaspoon coriander
- ½ teaspoon salt
- 1 daikon, chopped
- 1 cup of water

Method

1. Put all ingredients in the instant pot. Close and seal the lid.
2. After this, set the "Meat" mode and cook the stew for 35 minutes.
3. When the stew is cooked, carefully shred the meat with the help of the fork.

   Nutritional info per serve: calories 533, fat 28.8, fiber 0.5, carbs 1, protein 63.6

Fajita Pork Strips

Prep time: 5 minutes | **Cook time:** 45 minutes | **Yield:** 2 servings

Ingredients

- 11 oz pork shoulder, boneless, sliced
- 1 teaspoon fajita seasonings
- 2 tablespoons butter
- ½ cup of water

Method

1. Sprinkle the meat with fajita seasonings and put in the instant pot.
2. Add butter and cook it on saute mode for 5 minutes.
3. Then stir the pork strips and add water.
4. Seal the instant pot lid and set the "Manual" mode (High pressure).
5. Set timer for 40 minutes.
6. When the time is running out – make the natural pressure release for 10 minutes.

   Nutritional info per serve: calories 375, fat 29.9, fiber 0, carbs 0.7, protein 24.3

Poultry

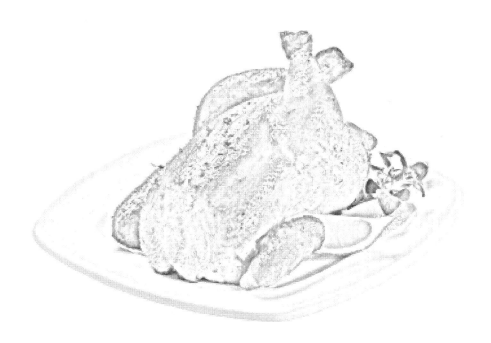

Garlic Chicken with Lemon

Prep time: 20 minutes | **Cook time:** 30 minutes | **Yield:** 6 servings

Ingredients

- 2-pound chicken thighs, skinless
- 1 tablespoon avocado oil
- 1 teaspoon minced garlic
- ½ teaspoon ground coriander
- 1 teaspoon lemon zest
- 1 teaspoon lemon juice
- 1/3 cup chicken broth
- 1 cup of water

Method

1. Pour water and insert the steamer rack in the instant pot. Pour water and chicken broth in the instant pot bowl.
2. Put the chicken thighs in the bowl and sprinkle them with avocado oil, minced garlic, ground coriander, lemon zest, and lemon juice.
3. Then shake the chicken thighs gently and transfer them on the steamer rack.
4. Close and seal the lid.
5. Cook the chicken for 15 minutes on manual mode (high pressure).
6. Then make a quick pressure release and transfer the chicken thighs on the plate.

   Nutritional info per serve: calories 294, fat 11.6, fiber 0.1, carbs 0.4, protein 44.1

Tuscan Chicken

Prep time: 15 minutes | **Cook time:** 12 minutes | **Yield:** 4 servings

Ingredients

- 4 chicken drumsticks
- 1 cup spinach, chopped
- 1 teaspoon minced garlic
- 1 teaspoon ground paprika
- 1 cup heavy cream
- 1 teaspoon cayenne pepper
- 1 oz sun-dried tomatoes, chopped

Method

1. Put all ingredients in the instant pot.
2. Close and seal the lid.
3. Cook the meal on manual mode (high pressure) for 12 minutes.
4. Then allow the natural pressure release for 10 minutes.
5. Serve the chicken with hot sauce from the instant pot.

   Nutritional info per serve: calories 188, fat 13.9, fiber 0.6, carbs 2.2, protein 13.7

Crack Chicken

Prep time: 15 minutes | **Cook time:** 20 minutes | **Yield:** 4 servings

Ingredients

- 1 cup chicken broth
- 1 teaspoon dried dill
- 1 teaspoon dried oregano
- ½ teaspoon onion powder
- 1-pound chicken breast, skinless, boneless
- ½ teaspoon salt
- 2 tablespoons mascarpone cheese
- 2 oz Cheddar cheese, shredded

Method

1. Pour the chicken broth in the instant pot.
2. Add dried ill, oregano, onion powder, chicken breast, and salt.
3. Close and seal the lid.
4. Cook the chicken breast on manual mode (high pressure) for 15 minutes.
5. Then make a quick pressure release and transfer the cooked chicken in the bowl.
6. Blend the chicken broth mixture with the help of the immersion blender.
7. Add mascarpone cheese and Cheddar cheese. Saute the liquid for 2 minutes on saute mode.
8. Meanwhile, shred the chicken.
9. Add it in the mascarpone mixture and mix it up. Saute the meal for 3 minutes more.

   Nutritional info per serve: calories 212, fat 8.9, fiber 0.2, carbs 1.3, protein 29.8

Thyme Chicken Gizzards

Prep time: 15 minutes | **Cook time:** 25 minutes | **Yield:** 4 servings

Ingredients

- 1-pound chicken gizzards, chopped
- 1 cup of water
- 1 teaspoon dried thyme
- 1 tablespoon butter
- 1 teaspoon salt
- ½ teaspoon peppercorns

Method

1. Put all ingredients in the instant pot.
2. Close and seal the lid.
3. Cook the chicken gizzards on manual mode (high pressure) for 25 minutes.
4. Allow the natural pressure release for 15 minutes before opening the lid.

   Nutritional info per serve: calories 50, fat 3.4, fiber 0.2, carbs 0.3, protein 4.5

White Chicken Chili

Prep time: 15 minutes | **Cook time:** 15 minutes | **Yield:** 4 servings

Ingredients

- 1 cup chicken broth
- 1-pound chicken fillet
- 1 teaspoon dried oregano
- ½ cup heavy cream
- 1 jalapeno, chopped
- 1 chili pepper, chopped
- 1 teaspoon cream cheese

Method

1. Put the chicken fillet in the instant pot.

2. Add chicken broth, oregano, heavy cream, jalapeno, and chili powder.

3. Cook the chicken on manual mode (high pressure) for 12 minutes. Make a quick pressure release and shred the chicken with the help of the fork.

4. Then add cream cheese and cook the chili on manual mode (high pressure) for 3 minutes. Allow the natural pressure release for 5 minutes.

   Nutritional info per serve: calories 282, fat 14.7, fiber 0.3, carbs 1.2, protein 34.5

Juicy Chicken Breast

Prep time: 10 minutes | **Cook time:** 15 minutes | **Yield:** 2 servings

Ingredients

- 8 oz chicken breast, skinless, boneless
- 1 cup of water
- ¼ cup butter
- 1 teaspoon chili flakes
- 1 teaspoon olive oil

Method

1. Heat up olive oil on saute mode for 2 minutes.

2. Then add the chicken breast and cook it for 3 minutes from each side.

3. Add water, butter, and chili flakes.

4. Close and seal the lid and cook the chicken for 10 minutes on High pressure.

5. Then make a quick pressure release and open the lid.

6. Slice the cooked chicken breast and sprinkle it with liquid from the instant pot.

   Nutritional info per serve: calories 353, fat 28.2, fiber 0, carbs 0.1, protein 24.3

Chicken in Gravy

Prep time: 10 minutes | **Cook time:** 15 minutes | **Yield:** 4 servings

Ingredients

- ¼ cup broccoli, chopped
- 2 oz celery stalk, chopped
- ¼ cup daikon, chopped
- 1 cup of water
- 4 chicken thighs
- 1 teaspoon salt
- 1 tablespoon coconut cream

Method

1. Put all ingredients in the instant pot and close the lid.

2. Cook the mixture for 15 minutes on manual mode (high pressure).

3. Then make a quick pressure release and open the lid.

4. Remove the chicken from the liquid.

5. Blend the liquid with the help of the immersion blender.

6. Then return the chicken thighs back in the blended sauce and saute the meal for 5 minutes.

   Nutritional info per serve: calories 293, fat 11.8, fiber 0.7, carbs 1.5, protein 42.8

Mustard Chicken Breast

Prep time: 10 minutes | **Cook time:** 15 minutes | **Yield:** 2 servings

Ingredients

- 10 oz chicken breast, boneless
- 1 tablespoon
- sunflower oil
- 2 teaspoons mustard
- 1 cup of water

Method

1. Pour water in the instant pot and insert the steamer rack.

2. In the shallow bowl, mix up sunflower oil and mustard.

3. Rub the chicken breast with mustard mixture and wrap in the foil.

4. Put the wrapped chicken on the steamer rack and close the lid.

5. Cook the meal in manual mode for 15 minutes. Make a quick pressure release.

   Nutritional info per serve: calories 239, fat 11.5, fiber 0.5, carbs 1.2, protein 30.9

Butter Chicken

Prep time: 10 minutes | **Cook time:** 20 minutes | **Yield:** 2 servings

Ingredients

- 8 oz chicken fillet, sliced
- 1 tomato, chopped
- 2 tablespoons mascarpone
- 1 teaspoon coconut
- oil
- 1 teaspoon ground paprika
- ½ teaspoon ground turmeric
- 1 tablespoon butter

Method

1. Rub the chicken fillet with ground paprika, ground turmeric, and paprika.
2. Put the sliced chicken in the instant pot.
3. Add tomato, mascarpone, coconut oil, and butter.
4. Close the lid and cook the meal on saute mode for 20 minutes.
5. Stir it every 5 minutes to avoid burning.

   Nutritional info per serve: calories 323, fat 18.7, fiber 0.9, carbs 2.6, protein 35.1

Parmesan Chicken Fillets

Prep time: 15 minutes | **Cook time:** 13 minutes | **Yield:** 2 servings

Ingredients

- 1 tomato, sliced
- 8 oz chicken fillets
- 2 oz Parmesan, sliced
- 1 teaspoon butter
- 4 tablespoons water
- 1 cup water, for cooking

Method

1. Pour water and insert the steamer rack in the instant pot.
2. Then grease the baking mold with butter.
3. Slice the chicken fillets into halves and put them in the mold.
4. Sprinkle the chicken with water and top with tomato and Parmesan.
5. Cover the baking mold with foil and place it on the rack.
6. Close and seal the lid.
7. Cook the meal in manual mode for 13 minutes. Then allow the natural pressure release for 10 minutes.

   Nutritional info per serve: calories 329, fat 16.4, fiber 0.4, carbs 2.2, protein 42.2

Chicken Alfredo

Prep time: 15 minutes | **Cook time:** 10 minutes | **Yield:** 4 servings

Ingredients

- ½ cup cremini mushrooms, sliced
- ¼ cup leek, chopped
- 1 tablespoon sesame oil
- 1 teaspoon chili flakes
- 1 cup heavy cream
- 1-pound chicken fillet, chopped
- 1 teaspoon Italian seasonings
- 1 tablespoon cream cheese

Method

1. Brush the instant pot boil with sesame oil from inside.
2. Put the chicken in the instant pot in one layer.
3. Then top it with mushrooms and leek.
4. Sprinkle the ingredients with chili flakes, heavy cream, Italian seasonings, and cream cheese.
5. Close and seal the lid.
6. Cook the meal on manual mode (high pressure) for 10 minutes.
7. When the time is finished, allow the natural pressure release for 10 minutes.

   Nutritional info per serve: calories 367, fat 24.2, fiber 0.2, carbs 2.2, protein 33.9

Paprika Chicken Wings

Prep time: 10 minutes | **Cook time:** 13 minutes | **Yield:** 4 servings

Ingredients

- 1-pound chicken wings, boneless
- 1 teaspoon ground paprika
- 1 teaspoon avocado
- oil
- ¼ teaspoon minced garlic
- ¾ cup beef broth

Method

1. Pour the avocado oil in the instant pot.
2. Rub the chicken wings with ground paprika and minced garlic and put them in the instant pot.
3. Cook the chicken on saute mode for 4 minutes from each side.
4. Then add beef broth and close the lid.
5. Saute the meal for 5 minutes more.

   Nutritional info per serve: calories 226, fat 8.9, fiber 0.3, carbs 0.6, protein 33.8

Cordon Bleu

Prep time: 20 minutes | **Cook time:** 7 minutes | **Yield:** 4 servings

Ingredients

- 1 cup coconut shred
- 4 deli ham slices
- 1-pound chicken breast, skinless, boneless
- 4 tablespoons butter, melted
- 1 teaspoon ground black pepper
- 4 Cheddar cheese slices
- 1 cup beef broth

Method

1. Cut the chicken breast into 4 fillets and beat them gently.

2. Then place the ham on the chicken fillets, add Cheddar cheese slices and roll them.

3. Mix up ground black pepper and melted butter.

4. Then dip the rolled chicken in the melted butter and coat in the coconut shred.

5. Pour beef broth and·insert the steamer rack in the instant pot.

6. Put the chicken on the steamer rack and close the lid.

7. Cook the meal on manual mode (high pressure) for 7 minutes.

8. Then allow the natural pressure release for 10 minutes.

   Nutritional info per serve: calories 601, fat 46.4, fiber 4.5, carbs 10, protein 37.1

Herbed Whole Chicken

Prep time: 20 minutes | **Cook time:** 25 minutes | **Yield:** 4 servings

Ingredients

- 1 ½ pound whole chicken
- 1 tablespoon poultry seasoning
- 2 tablespoons avocado oil
- 2 cups of water

Method

1. Pour water in the instant pot.

2. Then rub the chicken with poultry seasonings and avocado oil.

3. Put the chicken in the instant pot. Close and seal the lid.

4. Cook the meal in manual mode for 25 minutes.

5. When the time is finished, allow the natural pressure release for 10 minutes.

   Nutritional info per serve: calories 335, fat 13.6, fiber 0.4, carbs 1, protein 49.4

Chicken Pasta

Prep time: 10 minutes | **Cook time:** 20 minutes | **Yield:** 4 servings

Ingredients

- ¼ cup Monterey Jack cheese, shredded
- 1 tablespoon mascarpone cheese
- ½ cup coconut cream
- 1 teaspoon ground
- black pepper
- ½ teaspoon salt
- 1-pound chicken fillet, sliced
- 1 teaspoon olive oil

Method

1. Sprinkle the chicken fillet with ground black pepper and salt.

2. Then put it in the instant pot, add olive oil and cook on saute mode for 10 minutes.

3. Stir the chicken and add coconut cream and mascarpone cheese. Mix up well.

4. Add shredded cheese and close the lid.

5. Saute the chicken pasta for 10 minutes on saute mode.

6. Stir the cooked chicken pasta well before serving.

   Nutritional info per serve: calories 329, fat 19.4, fiber 0.8, carbs 2.2, protein 35.7

Pulled Chicken

Prep time: 10 minutes | **Cook time:** 12 minutes | **Yield:** 2 servings

Ingredients

- ¼ teaspoon smoked paprika
- ½ teaspoon ground cumin
- 3 tablespoons sugar-
- free ketchup
- 1 cup of water
- 1 teaspoon Erythritol
- 10 oz chicken fillet

Method

1. Put all the ingredients in the instant pot. Close and seal the lid.

2. Cook the meal on Manual (high pressure) for 12 minutes.

3. Then make a quick pressure release and open the lid.

4. Shred the chicken with the help of 2 forks and transfer in the serving bowls.

5. Add ½ part of the remaining liquid from the instant pot.

   Nutritional info per serve: calories 280, fat 10.7, fiber 0.2, carbs 7.4, protein 41.1

Fiesta Chicken

Prep time: 20 minutes | **Cook time:** 15 minutes | **Yield:** 4 servings

Ingredients

- 1 cup cauliflower, shredded
- 1 teaspoon taco seasonings
- ¼ cup bell pepper, chopped
- 1 tomato, chopped
- 1 cup chicken broth
- ½ teaspoon chili flakes
- 1 tablespoon butter

1-pound chicken thighs, skinless, boneless, chopped

Method

1. Melt the butter in the instant pot on saute mode.
2. After this, add bell pepper, tomato, and cauliflower.
3. Sprinkle the vegetables with taco seasonings and cook them for 10 minutes on saute mode.
4. After this, add chicken thighs, chili flakes, and chicken broth.
5. Close and seal the lid and cook the meal on manual mode (high pressure) for 15 minutes.
6. Allow the natural pressure release for 10 minutes.

Nutritional info per serve: calories 265, fat 11.7, fiber 3.2, carbs 0.9, protein 34.8

Chicken Masala

Prep time: 10 minutes | **Cook time:** 17 minutes | **Yield:** 3 servings

Ingredients

- 12 oz chicken fillet
- 1 tablespoon masala spices
- 1 tablespoon avocado oil
- 3 tablespoons organic almond milk

Method

1. Heat up avocado oil in the instant pot on saute mode for 2 minutes.
2. Meanwhile, chop the chicken fillet roughly and mix it up with masala spices.
3. Add almond milk and transfer the chicken in the instant pot.
4. Cook the chicken bites on saute mode for 15 minutes. Stir the meal occasionally.

Nutritional info per serve: calories 211, fat 8.6, fiber 0.2, carbs 6.2, protein 25.4

Sesame Chicken

Prep time: 15 minutes | **Cook time:** 12 minutes | **Yield:** 2 servings

Ingredients

- ½ teaspoon of five spices
- ½ teaspoon sesame seeds
- ½ cup broccoli, chopped
- 6 oz chicken fillet,
- sliced
- ½ cup chicken broth
- 1 teaspoon coconut aminos
- 1 tablespoon avocado oil

Method

1. In the mixing bowl, mix up avocado oil, coconut aminos, and sesame seeds.
2. Add five spices.
3. After this, mix up sliced chicken fillet and coconut aminos mixture.
4. Put the chicken in the instant pot. Add chicken broth and broccoli.
5. Close and seal the lid.
6. Cook the meal on manual mode (high pressure) for 12 minutes. Make a quick pressure release.

Nutritional info per serve: calories 195, fat 8, fiber 1, carbs 2.8, protein 26.7

Chicken Curry with Cilantro

Prep time: 15 minutes | **Cook time:** 12 minutes | **Yield:** 4 servings

Ingredients

- 1 eggplant, chopped
- ¼ cup fresh cilantro, chopped
- 1 teaspoon curry powder
- 1 cup coconut cream
- 1 teaspoon coconut oil
- 1-pound chicken breast, skinless, boneless, cubed

Method

1. Put the coconut oil and chicken breast in the instant pot.
2. Saute the ingredients on saute mode for 5 minutes.
3. Then stir well and add cilantro, eggplant, coconut cream, and curry powder.
4. Close and seal the lid.
5. Cook the meal on manual mode (high pressure) for 7 minutes.
6. Make a quick pressure release and transfer the cooked chicken in the serving bowls.

Nutritional info per serve: calories 308, fat 18.6, fiber 5.6, carbs 10.4, protein 26.6

Tender Chicken Thighs

Prep time: 10 minutes | **Cook time:** 16 minutes | **Yield:** 4 servings

Ingredients

- 1 teaspoon dried sage
- 1 teaspoon ground turmeric
- 2 teaspoons avocado oil
- 4 chicken thighs, skinless
- 1 cup of water
- 1 teaspoon sesame oil

Method

1. Rub the chicken thighs with dried sage, ground turmeric, sesame oil, and avocado oil.

2. Then pour water in the instant pot and insert the steamer rack.

3. Place the chicken thighs on the rack and close the lid.

4. Cook the meal on manual (high pressure) for 16 minutes.

5. Then make a quick pressure release and open the lid.

6. Let the cooked chicken thighs cool for 10 minutes before serving.

    Nutritional info per serve: calories 293, fat 12.3, fiber 0.3, carbs 0.6, protein 42.3

Chicken Nuggets

Prep time: 10 minutes | **Cook time:** 9 minutes | **Yield:** 5 servings

Ingredients

- 8 oz chicken fillet
- 1 teaspoon ground turmeric
- ½ teaspoon ground
- coriander
- ½ cup almond flour
- 2 eggs, beaten
- ½ cup butter

Method

1. Chop the chicken fillet roughly into the medium size pieces.

2. In the mixing bowl, mix up ground turmeric, ground coriander, and almond flour.

3. Then dip the chicken pieces in the beaten egg and coat in the almond flour mixture.

4. Toss the butter in the instant pot and melt it on saute mode for 4 minutes.

5. Then put the coated chicken in the hot butter and cook for 5 minutes or until the nuggets are golden brown.

    Nutritional info per serve: calories 343, fat 28.9, fiber 1.3, carbs 2.8, protein 18

Chicken Jalapenos Roll

Prep time: 15 minutes | **Cook time:** 20 minutes | **Yield:** 4 servings

Ingredients

- 16 oz chicken fillet
- 2 jalapenos, trimmed, seeded
- 1 tablespoon olive oil
- 1 teaspoon Italian seasoning
- 1 teaspoon ground paprika
- ½ teaspoon salt
- 2 Cheddar cheese slices
- 1 cup water, for cooking

Method

1. Beat the chicken fillet with the help of the kitchen hammer.

2. Then sprinkle it with Italian seasonings, ground paprika, and salt.

3. After this, put the cheese on the fillet. Add jalapenos and roll the chicken fillet into a roll.

4. Brush it with the help of the olive oil and put it in the baking pan.

5. Pour water and insert the steamer rack in the instant pot.

6. Put the baking pan with chicken on the steamer rack. Close and seal the lid.

7. Cook the meal on manual (high pressure) for 20 minutes. Make a quick pressure release.

    Nutritional info per serve: calories 309, fat 17, fiber 0.4, carbs 1, protein 36.5

Smoky Chicken Breast

Prep time: 10 minutes | **Cook time:** 75 minutes | **Yield:** 4 servings

Ingredients

- 1-pound chicken breast, skinless, boneless
- 1 tablespoon Keto
- ketchup
- 1 teaspoon Erythritol
- 1 teaspoon allspices
- 1 cup chicken broth

Method

1. Put all ingredients in the instant pot.

2. Close the lid and cook the ingredients on Meat/Stew mode for 75 minutes.

3. When the cooking time is finished, open the lid and shred the chicken breast.

4. Stir the meal well before serving.

    Nutritional info per serve: calories 144, fat 3.2, fiber 0.1, carbs 2.8, protein 25.4

Fajita Strips

Prep time: 10 minutes | **Cook time:** 25 minutes | **Yield:** 4 servings

Ingredients

- 1 bell pepper, cut into strips
- 2 oz scallions, chopped
- 1 teaspoon Fajita seasonings
- 15 oz chicken fillet, cut into strips
- 1 teaspoon coconut oil
- ½ teaspoon ginger paste

Method

1. Heat up coconut oil on saute mode for 3 minutes.
2. Add scallions and bell pepper strips.
3. Saute them for 5 minutes.
4. After this, add Fajita seasonings, chicken strips, and ginger paste.
5. Close the lid and cook the meal for 15 minutes. Stir the chicken from time to time during cooking.

   Nutritional info per serve: calories 229, fat 9.1, fiber 0.8, carbs 4, protein 31.3

Greek Burger

Prep time: 15 minutes | **Cook time:** 20 minutes | **Yield:** 2 servings

Ingredients

- 1 cup ground chicken
- 1 tablespoon lemon juice
- 2 tablespoons coconut flour
- ½ teaspoon minced garlic
- ½ teaspoon dried parsley
- 1 cup water, for cooking

Method

1. In the mixing bowl, mix up ground chicken, lemon juice, coconut flour, minced garlic, and dried parsley.
2. Make 2 burgers and place them in the baking pan.
3. Pour water and insert the steamer rack in the instant pot.
4. Then place the pan with burgers on the steamer. Close and seal the lid.
5. Cook the meal on manual mode (high pressure) for 20 minutes. Allow the natural pressure release for 10 minutes.

   Nutritional info per serve: calories 173, fat 6.5, fiber 3.1, carbs 5.1, protein 21.9

Dijon Turkey Meatballs

Prep time: 15 minutes | **Cook time:** 14 minutes | **Yield:** 4 servings

Ingredients

- 14 oz ground turkey
- 1 tablespoon Dijon mustard
- ½ cup coconut flour
- 1 teaspoon onion powder
- 1 teaspoon salt
- ½ cup chicken broth
- 1 tablespoon avocado oil

Method

1. In the mixing bowl, mix up ground turkey, Dijon mustard, coconut flour, onion powder, and salt.
2. Make the meatballs with the help of the fingertips.
3. Then pour avocado oil in the instant pot and heat it up for1 minute.
4. Add the meatballs and cook them for 2 minutes from each side.
5. Then add chicken broth. Close and seal the lid.
6. Cook the meatballs for 10 minutes. Make a quick pressure release.

   Nutritional info per serve: calories 268, fat 13.2, fiber 6.3, carbs 11, protein 30

Tender Turkey Tetrazzini

Prep time: 15 minutes | **Cook time:** 20 minutes | **Yield:** 4 servings

Ingredients

- 14 oz turkey, breast, cooked, shredded
- ½ cup mushrooms, sliced
- 2 oz Parmesan, grated
- 1 cup spaghetti squash, chopped, cooked
- 2 tablespoons butter, melted
- ½ cup heavy cream
- ½ cup Mozzarella, shredded
- ½ cup of water

Method

1. Put shredded turkey, mushrooms, Parmesan, and spaghetti squash in the instant pot. Mix up well.
2. In the mixing bowl, mix up butter, heavy cream, Mozzarella, and water.
3. Pour the liquid over the turkey.
4. Close and seal the lid.
5. Cook the meal on manual mode (high pressure) for 20 minutes. Allow the natural pressure release for 10 minutes.

   Nutritional info per serve: calories 337, fat 20.1, fiber 0.1, carbs 3.1, protein 35.4

Cheese Chicken Kofte

Prep time: 10 minutes | **Cook time:** 10 minutes | **Yield:** 4 servings

Ingredients

- 1 ½ cup ground chicken
- 1 teaspoon chili flakes
- 1 teaspoon garlic powder
- ½ cup Cheddar cheese, shredded
- 1 egg, beaten
- 3 tablespoons coconut flour
- 1 tablespoon coconut oil

Method

1. In the mixing bowl, mix up ground chicken, chili flakes, garlic powder, shredded cheese, egg, and coconut flour.
2. Then make the small meatballs and press them gently with the help of the hand palm.
3. Heat up coconut oil on saute mode for 2 minutes.
4. Then put the chicken kofte inside the instant pot in one layer and cook them for 4 minutes from each side.

Nutritional info per serve: calories 227, fat 13.6, fiber 2.3, carbs 4.5, protein 21

Chicken with Pizza Stuffing

Prep time: 20 minutes | **Cook time:** 12 minutes | **Yield:** 4 servings

Ingredients

- 12 oz chicken fillet
- 3 oz ground sausages
- ½ bell pepper, chopped
- ½ teaspoon chili flakes
- ¼ cup Cheddar cheese, shredded
- ½ tomato, chopped
- 1 teaspoon Italian seasonings
- 1 cup water, for cooking

Method

1. In the mixing bowl, mix up ground sausages, bell pepper, chili flakes, Cheddar cheese, tomato, and Italian seasonings.
2. Then make the cut (pocket) in the chicken fillet and fill it with ground sausages mixture.
3. Wrap the chicken in the foil and place it on the steamer rack.
4. Pour water and transfer the steamer rack in the instant pot.
5. Cook the meal on manual mode (high pressure) for 22 minutes. Allow the natural pressure release for 10 minutes.

Nutritional info per serve: calories 272, fat 15.1, fiber 0.3, carbs 1.7, protein 30.7

Poblano Chicken Strips

Prep time: 10 minutes | **Cook time:** 29 minutes | **Yield:** 4 servings

Ingredients

- 2 Poblano peppers, sliced
- 16 oz chicken fillet
- ½ teaspoon salt
- ½ cup coconut cream
- 1 tablespoon butter
- ½ teaspoon chili powder

Method

1. Heat up the butter on saute mode for 3 minutes.
2. Add Poblano and cook them for 3 minutes.
3. Meanwhile, cut the chicken fillet into the strips and sprinkle with salt and chili powder.
4. Add the chicken strips to the instant pot.
5. Then add coconut cream and close the lid.
6. Cook the meal on saute mode for 20 minutes.

Nutritional info per serve: calories 320, fat 18.5, fiber 1.1, carbs 4, protein 34

Philadelphia Stuffed Chicken Breast

Prep time: 10 minutes | **Cook time:** 16 minutes | **Yield:** 5 servings

Ingredients

- 1-pound chicken breast, skinless, boneless
- 2 tablespoons cream cheese
- 1 tablespoon chives, chopped
- ½ teaspoon minced garlic
- ½ teaspoon salt
- 1 tablespoon avocado oil
- 1 cup water, for cooking

Method

1. Make the cut in the shape of the pocket in the chicken breast. Rub the chicken with salt.
2. After this, in the mixing bowl, mix up cream cheese, chives, and minced garlic.
3. Rub the chicken breast with salt and fill with the cream cheese.
4. Then secure the "chicken pocket" with the help of the toothpicks.
5. Pour water and insert the steamer rack in the instant pot.
6. Then put the chicken breast in the baking pan and transfer it on the rack.
7. Cook the meal on manual mode (high pressure) for 25 minutes. Allow the natural pressure release for 10 minutes.

Nutritional info per serve: calories 122, fat 4, fiber 0.2, carbs 0.4, protein 19.6

Chicken Fingers

Prep time: 10 minutes | **Cook time:** 7 minutes | **Yield:** 4 servings

Ingredients

- 2 eggs, beaten
- 1 tablespoon coconut cream
- ½ teaspoon ground paprika
- ½ teaspoon ground turmeric
- ½ teaspoon salt
- ½ cup almond flour
- 1-pound chicken fillet
- 1 tablespoon coconut oil

Method

1. Cut the chicken fillet on the strips and sprinkle with salt, ground paprika, and ground turmeric.
2. In the mixing bowl, mix up coconut cream and eggs.
3. Then dip the chicken strips in the egg mixture. After this, coat the chicken in the almond flour.
4. Repeat the steps one more time.
5. Then preheat the coconut oil on saute mode for 2 minutes and put the chicken strips inside in one layer.
6. Cook the chicken strips on saute mode for 3 minutes from each side.

   Nutritional info per serve: calories 371, fat 21.6, fiber 1.7, carbs 3.7, protein 38.7

Spanish Chicken

Prep time: 10 minutes | **Cook time:** 25 minutes | **Yield:** 4 servings

Ingredients

- 4 chicken thighs, skinless
- 1 teaspoon tomato paste
- 2 oz olives, sliced
- ½ cup chicken broth
- 1 teaspoon dried oregano
- 1 tablespoon goat milk butter

Method

1. Put the goat milk butter in the instant pot and heat it up on saute mode for 2 minutes.
2. Then add chicken thighs and cook them for 4 minutes from each side.
3. Add dried oregano, olives, tomato paste, and chicken broth.
4. Close and seal the lid and cook the Spanish chicken on manual mode (high pressure) for 15 minutes.
5. Make a quick pressure release.

   Nutritional info per serve: calories 328, fat 15.6, fiber 0.7, carbs 1.5, protein 43.1

Chicken Lombardy

Prep time: 15 minutes | **Cook time:** 30 minutes | **Yield:** 4 servings

Ingredients

- 4 chicken thighs
- 1 oz butter
- ½ teaspoon garam masala
- ¼ cup apple cider vinegar
- 2 tablespoons coconut flour
- 3 oz Parmesan, grated
- ½ cup of water
- 1 oz Mozzarella cheese, shredded

Method

1. Heat up butter on saute mode.
2. When the butter is melted, add chicken thighs and sprinkle them with garam masala. Cook them for 3 minutes from each side.
3. After this, add apple cider vinegar, coconut flour, and ½ cup water.
4. Close and seal the lid and cook the chicken on manual (high pressure) for 15 minutes.
5. Allow the natural pressure release for 10 minutes.
6. Then top the chicken with all cheese and saute for 5 minutes more.

   Nutritional info per serve: calories 435, fat 22.7, fiber 1.5, carbs 3.7, protein 51.6

Mushroom Mini Pizza

Prep time: 10 minutes | **Cook time:** 10 minutes | **Yield:** 4 servings

Ingredients

- 4 Portobello mushroom caps
- 2 oz Parmesan, grated
- ½ tomato, chopped
- 2 oz ground chicken
- 1 cup water, for cooking

Method

1. Pour water and insert the steamer rack in the instant pot.
2. Then fill the mushroom caps with chopped tomato, ground chicken, and grated Parmesan.
3. Place the mushroom caps on the rack. Close and seal the lid.
4. Cook the mini pizzas on manual mode (high pressure) for 10 minutes.
5. Then make a quick pressure release and transfer the mini pizzas on the big serving plate.

   Nutritional info per serve: calories 81, fat 4.2, fiber 0.5, carbs 2.2, protein 9.4

Provolone Stuffed Chicken

Prep time: 15 minutes | **Cook time:** 20 minutes | **Yield:** 4 servings

Ingredients

- 12 oz chicken fillet
- 4 oz provolone cheese, sliced
- 1 tablespoon cream cheese
- ½ teaspoon dried cilantro
- ½ teaspoon smoked paprika
- 1 cup water, for cooking

Method

1. Beat the chicken fillet well and rub it with dried cilantro and smoked paprika.

2. Then spread it with cream cheese and top with Provolone cheese.

3. Roll the chicken fillet into the roll and wrap in the foil.

4. Pour water and insert the rack in the instant pot.

5. Place the chicken roll on the rack. Close and seal the lid.

6. Cook it on manual mode (high pressure) for 20 minutes.

7. Make a quick pressure release and slice the chicken roll into the servings.

Nutritional info per serve: calories 271, fat 14.8, fiber 0.1, carbs 0.8, protein 32.1

Hot BBQ Wings

Prep time: 10 minutes | **Cook time:** 30 minutes | **Yield:** 6 servings

Ingredients

- 1-pound chicken wings
- 1 teaspoon keto ketchup
- ½ cup keto BBQ sauce
- 1 tablespoon avocado oil
- ¼ cup of water

Method

1. Heat up avocado oil in the instant pot on saute mode.

2. Add chicken wings and cook them for 2 minutes from each side.

3. After this, add all remaining ingredients. Close the lid.

4. Saute the chicken wings for 25 minutes.

Nutritional info per serve: calories 179, fat 6, fiber 0.2, carbs 7.9, protein 21.9

Vinegar Chicken Fillets

Prep time: 15 minutes | **Cook time:** 25 minutes | **Yield:** 4 servings

Ingredients

- 1 teaspoon Cajun seasonings
- ¼ cup apple cider vinegar
- 1-pound chicken fillet
- 1 tablespoon sesame oil
- ¼ cup of water

Method

1. Put all ingredients in the instant pot. Close and seal the lid.

2. Cook the chicken fillets on manual mode (high pressure) for 25 minutes.

3. Allow the natural pressure release for 10 minutes.

Nutritional info per serve: calories 249, fat 11.8, fiber 0, carbs 0.1, protein 32.8

Chicken Shawarma

Prep time: 15 minutes | **Cook time:** 17 minutes | **Yield:** 4 servings

Ingredients

- 1-pound chicken fillet
- ½ teaspoon ground coriander
- ½ teaspoon smoked paprika
- ½ teaspoon dried thyme
- 1 tablespoon tahini sauce
- 1 teaspoon lemon juice
- 1 teaspoon heavy cream
- 1 cup water, for cooking

Method

1. Rub the chicken fillet with ground coriander, smoked paprika, thyme, and wrap in the foil.

2. Then pour water and insert the steamer rack in the instant pot.

3. Place the wrapped chicken in the steamer; close and seal the lid.

4. Cook the chicken on manual mode (high pressure) for 17 minutes. Make a quick pressure release.

5. Make the sauce: mix up heavy cream, lemon juice, and tahini paste.

6. Slice the chicken and sprinkle it with sauce.

Nutritional info per serve: calories 234, fat 10, fiber 0.2, carbs 0.8, protein 33.4

Pecan Chicken

Prep time: 10 minutes | **Cook time:** 15 minutes | **Yield:** 2 servings

Ingredients

- 6 oz chicken fillet, cubed
- 2 pecans, chopped
- 1 teaspoon coconut aminos
- ½ bell pepper, chopped
- 1 tablespoon coconut oil
- ¼ cup apple cider vinegar
- ¼ cup chicken broth

Method

1. Melt coconut oil on saute mode and add chicken cubes.
2. Add bell pepper, and pecans.
3. Saute the ingredients for 10 minutes and add apple cider vinegar, chicken broth, and coconut aminos.
4. Saute the chicken for 5 minutes more.

Nutritional info per serve: calories 341, fat 23.4, fiber 1.9, carbs 5.1, protein 27

Pancetta Wings

Prep time: 15 minutes | **Cook time:** 7 minutes | **Yield:** 4 servings

Ingredients

- 4 chicken wings
- 2 oz pancetta, sliced
- 1 teaspoon ground black pepper
- ½ teaspoon salt
- 1 cup water, for cooking

Method

1. Put the sliced pancetta in the baking pan in one layer.
2. Then sprinkle the chicken wings with ground black pepper and salt and place them over the pancetta.
3. Cover the chicken with foil.
4. After this, pour water and insert the steamer rack in the instant pot.
5. Put the baking pan with chicken on the rack. Close and seal the lid.
6. Cook the chicken wings on manual mode (high pressure) for 7 minutes. Then allow the natural pressure release for 10 minutes.

Nutritional info per serve: calories 177, fat 12.6, fiber 0.1, carbs 0.5, protein 14.4

Chicken Slaw Mix

Prep time: 10 minutes | **Cook time:** 15 minutes | **Yield:** 2 servings

Ingredients

- ½ cup slaw mix
- 1 tablespoon heavy cream
- 6 oz chicken, chopped
- 1 teaspoon ground black pepper
- 1 tablespoon olive oil
- 1 teaspoon lemon juice

Method

1. Put the chicken in the instant pot and sprinkle with lemon juice, ground black pepper, and olive oil.
2. Stir gently and cook it on saute mode for 15 minutes. Stir it from time to time.
3. Then cool the cooked chicken gently and mix it up with slaw mix.
4. Add heavy cream and mix up well.

Nutritional info per serve: calories 236, fat 12.4, fiber 0.3, carbs 5.5, protein 25.1

Low Carb Pot Pie

Prep time: 15 minutes | **Cook time:** 50 minutes | **Yield:** 6 servings

Ingredients

- 10 oz chicken fillet, chopped
- 1 teaspoon salt
- ½ teaspoon ground black pepper
- ½ cup heavy cream
- 2 tablespoons scallions, chopped
- 1 daikon, diced
- ½ cup Mozzarella, shredded
- ½ cup coconut flour
- 2 eggs, beaten
- Cooking spray
- 1 cup water, for cooking

Method

1. Put chicken, salt, water, and ground black pepper in the instant pot.
2. Close and seal the lid and cook the chicken for 30 minutes on manual mode (high pressure). Make a quick pressure release.
3. Meanwhile, spray the pan with cooking spray and heat it up. Add scallions and daikon and roast the vegetables for 5 minutes.
4. Put the cooked vegetables in the round pan (pot pie pan).
5. Add cooked chicken and heavy cream.
6. Mix up Mozzarella, coconut flour, and eggs.
7. Top the chicken with cheese mixture and bake in the oven for 20 minutes at 390F.

Nutritional info per serve: calories 202, fat 10.9, fiber 4.3, carbs 7.1, protein 18.6

Club Salad

Prep time: 15 minutes | **Cook time:** 25 minutes | **Yield:** 2 servings

Ingredients

- ½ cup butter leaves lettuce, chopped
- 1 oz bacon, chopped cooked
- 5 oz chicken fillet, chopped
- 1 avocado slice, chopped
- 1 tablespoon keto mayonnaise
- 1 cup water, for cooking

Method

1. Pour water in the instant pot. Add chicken and cook it on manual mode (high pressure) for 25 minutes. Make a quick pressure release.
2. Chop the cooked chicken and put it in the salad bowl.
3. Add bacon, lettuce, avocado, and shake well.
4. Sprinkle the salad with keto mayonnaise.

Nutritional info per serve: calories 237, fat 13.7, fiber 0.1, carbs 1.2, protein 25.9

Chicken&Cheddar Biscuits

Prep time: 15 minutes | **Cook time:** 10 minutes | **Yield:** 4 servings

Ingredients

- 3 oz chicken fillet, cooked, shredded
- 2 tablespoons almond flour
- 1 egg, beaten
- ½ teaspoon minced
- garlic
- ¼ cup coconut cream
- 3 oz Cheddar cheese, shredded
- 1 cup water, for cooking

Method

1. In the mixing bowl, mix up shredded chicken, almond flour, egg, minced garlic, coconut cream, and shredded cheese.
2. Then transfer the homogenous mixture in the muffin molds and flatten them gently with the help of the spoon.
3. Pour water and insert the steamer rack in the instant pot.
4. Place the muffin molds on the rack. Close and seal the lid.
5. Cook the meal on manual mode (high pressure) for 10 minutes. Allow the natural pressure release for 10 minutes.

Nutritional info per serve: calories 257, fat 20.3, fiber 1.8, carbs 4.3, protein 16.2

Bacon-Wrapped Tenders

Prep time: 15 minutes | **Cook time:** 15 minutes | **Yield:** 2 servings

Ingredients

- 4 oz chicken fillet
- 2 bacon slices
- ½ teaspoon ground paprika
- ¼ teaspoon salt
- 1 teaspoon olive oil
- 1 cup water, for cooking

Method

1. Cut the chicken fillet on 2 tenders and sprinkle them with salt, ground paprika, and olive oil.
2. Wrap the chicken tenders in the bacon and transfer in the steamer rack,
3. Pour water and insert the steamer rack with the chicken tenders in the instant pot.
4. Close and seal the lid and cook the meal on manual mode (high pressure) for 15 minutes.
5. When the time is finished, allow the natural pressure release for 10 minutes.

Nutritional info per serve: calories 232, fat 14.5, fiber 0.2, carbs 0.6, protein 23.5

TSO Chicken Drumsticks

Prep time: 10 minutes | **Cook time:** 20 minutes | **Yield:** 6 servings

Ingredients

- 6 chicken thighs
- 1 tablespoon apple cider vinegar
- 1 tablespoon coconut aminos
- ½ teaspoon ginger,
- grated
- 1 teaspoon Splenda
- ½ teaspoon chili flakes
- ¼ cup avocado oil
- 1/3 cup water

Method

1. Heat up avocado oil on saute mode for 3 minutes and add chicken thighs.
2. Saute the chicken for 6 minutes.
3. Then add the rest of the ingredients and stir them gently.
4. Close and seal the lid and cook the meal on Poultry mode for 10 minutes.
5. Carefully stir the cooked chicken.

Nutritional info per serve: calories 179, fat 11.2, fiber 0.4, carbs 1.8, protein 19.1

Chicken Divan

Prep time: 15 minutes | **Cook time:** 10 minutes | **Yield:** 4 servings

Ingredients

- 1 cup broccoli, chopped
- 2 tablespoons cream cheese
- ½ cup heavy cream
- 1 tablespoon curry powder
- ¼ cup chicken broth
- ½ cup Cheddar cheese, grated
- 6 oz chicken fillet, cooked chopped

Method

1. Mix up broccoli and curry powder and put the mixture in the instant pot.
2. Add heavy cream and cream cheese.
3. Then add chicken and mix up the ingredients.
4. Then add chicken broth and heavy cream.
5. Top the mixture with Cheddar cheese. Close and seal the lid.
6. Cook the meal on manual mode (high pressure) for 10 minutes. Allow the natural pressure release for 5 minutes, open the lid and cool the meal for 10 minutes.

Nutritional info per serve: calories 222, fat 15.5, fiber 1.1, carbs 3.2, protein 17.7

Chicken Zucchini Rings

Prep time: 15 minutes | **Cook time:** 20 minutes | **Yield:** 2 servings

Ingredients

- 1 zucchini, trimmed
- 6 oz ground chicken
- ½ teaspoon chili flakes
- ½ teaspoon salt
- ½ teaspoon ginger paste
- 1 cup keto marinara sauce

Method

1. Slice the zucchini into the thick rings and remove the zucchini meat from the ring.
2. In the mixing bowl, mix up ground chicken, chili flakes, salt, and ginger paste.
3. Then fill the zucchini rings with chicken mixture and place them in the instant pot.
4. Add marinara sauce, close and seal the lid.
5. Cook the meal on manual mode (high pressure) for 20 minutes. Make a quick pressure release.

Nutritional info per serve: calories 203, fat 7.5, fiber 1.7, carbs 7.1, protein 26.3

Chicken Fritters

Prep time: 10 minutes | **Cook time:** 10 minutes | **Yield:** 4 servings

Ingredients

- 1 zucchini, grated
- 1 cup ground chicken
- 1 teaspoon chili powder
- 1 tablespoon avocado oil
- 1 egg, beaten

Method

1. Mix up zucchini, ground chicken, chili powder, and egg. When the mixture is smooth, make the medium size fritters.
2. Heat up the avocado oil in the instant pot on saute mode (appx. for 3 minutes).
3. Place the chicken fritters in the hot oil and cook them for 5 minutes per side.

Nutritional info per serve: calories 97, fat 4.3, fiber 0.9, carbs 2.3, protein 12.2

Chicken Carbonara

Prep time: 15 minutes | **Cook time:** 25minutes | **Yield:** 5 servings

Ingredients

- 1-pound chicken, skinless, boneless, chopped
- 1 cup heavy cream
- 1 cup spinach, chopped
- 2 oz Parmesan, grated
- 1 teaspoon ground black pepper
- 1 tablespoon coconut oil
- 2 oz bacon, chopped

Method

1. Put the coconut oil and chopped chicken in the instant pot.
2. Saute the chicken for 10 minutes. Stir it from time to time.
3. Then add ground black pepper, and spinach. Stir the mixture well and saute for 5 minutes more.
4. Then add heavy cream and Parmesan. Close and seal the lid.
5. Cook the meal on manual mode (high pressure) for 10 minutes. Allow the natural pressure release for 10 minutes.

Nutritional info per serve: calories 343, fat 21.6, fiber 0.2, carbs 1.7, protein 34.8

Crackle Chicken

Prep time: 10 minutes | **Cook time:** 30 minutes | **Yield:** 2 servings

Ingredients

- 2 chicken thighs
- 4 tablespoons butter
- ½ teaspoon white pepper
- ½ teaspoon salt
- 1 cup water, for cooking

Method

1. Pour water in the instant pot and add chicken thighs.

2. Close and seal the lid and cook the chicken for 20 minutes on manual mode (high pressure). Make a quick pressure release.

3. Remove the chicken and clean the instant pot.

4. Then toss the butter in the instant pot and melt it on saute mode.

5. Sprinkle the chicken thigs with salt and white pepper and add them in the melted butter.

6. Saute the chicken for 5 minutes per side.

Nutritional info per serve: calories 365, fat 33.1, fiber 0.1, carbs 0.4, protein 19.3

Marry Me Chicken

Prep time: 15 minutes | **Cook time:** 25 minutes | **Yield:** 4 servings

Ingredients

- 4 chicken thighs
- 1 teaspoon olive oil
- 1 teaspoon garlic, diced
- 1 teaspoon dried thyme
- 1 tablespoon avocado
- oil
- ¼ cup chicken broth
- ½ cup heavy cream
- 1 teaspoon salt
- 1 teaspoon ground black pepper

Method

1. Pour olive oil in the instant pot and add chicken thighs.

2. Saute them for 4 minutes from each side. Sprinkle the chicken with salt and ground black pepper.

3. Then transfer the chicken on the plate.

4. Add avocado oil in the instant pot.

5. Then add dried thyme and garlic. Saute the ingredients for 2 minutes. Add chicken thighs, chicken broth, and heavy cream. Saute the chicken for 15 minutes.

Nutritional info per serve: calories 232, fat 17.3, fiber 0.4, carbs 1.4, protein 19.8

Feta Chicken Drumsticks

Prep time: 7 minutes | **Cook time:** 15 minutes | **Yield:** 2 servings

Ingredients

- 4 lemon slices
- 2 chicken thighs
- 1 tablespoon Greek seasoning
- 4 oz Feta, crumbled
- 1 teaspoon butter
- ½ cup of water

Method

1. Rub the chicken thighs with Greek seasoning.

2. Then spread the chicken with butter.

3. Pour water in the instant pot and place the trivet.

4. Place the chicken on the foil and top with the lemon slices. Top it with Feta.

5. Wrap the chicken in the foil and transfer on the trivet.

6. Cook on the "Saute" mode for 10 minutes. Then make a quick pressure release for 5 minutes.

7. Discard the foil from the chicken thighs and serve!

Nutritional info per serve: calories 341, fat 24.2, fiber 0.4, carbs 5.9, protein 27.5

Chicken Cubes in Succulent Sauce

Prep time: 10 minutes | **Cook time:** 25 minutes | **Yield:** 2 servings

Ingredients

- 14 oz chicken breast
- ½ teaspoon ground cardamom
- ¼ teaspoon ground coriander
- ¾ teaspoon minced garlic
- ½ cup of coconut milk
- ½ teaspoon salt
- ¾ teaspoon nutmeg
- 1 teaspoon almond butter

Method

1. Mix up together the ground cardamom, ground coriander, minced garlic, and nutmeg.

2. Then chop the chicken breast roughly.

3. Stir the spice mixture in the full-fat cream and whisk until homogenous.

4. Place the almond butter and chicken in the instant pot bowl.

5. Add coconut milk and lock the instant pot lid.

6. Cook on the "Saute" mode for 25 minutes.

Nutritional info per serve: calories 421, fat 24.1, fiber 2.5, carbs 5.9, protein 45.3

Celery Salad with Chicken

Prep time: 5 minutes | **Cook time:** 6 minutes | **Yield:** 2 servings

Ingredients

- 1 cup celery, raw, diced
- 5 oz chicken breast, chopped
- 1 tablespoon butter
- 1 tablespoon lemon juice
- ½ teaspoon chili flakes
- 1 tablespoon fresh dill, chopped
- ½ tomato, chopped
- ¾ cup of water

Method

1. Toss the butter in the instant pot and preheat it on the "Saute" mode.
2. Add chopped chicken breast. Sprinkle it with the chili flakes and cook for 4 minutes.
3. Add water and close the lid. Seal the lid and set the "Manual" mode + press timer for 3 minutes (High Pressure). Make the quick pressure release then.
4. Add tomato and celery in the salad bowl.
5. Add fresh dill and lemon juice.
6. After this, add chicken breast (don't use the chicken water).
7. Stir the salad directly before serving.

Nutritional info per serve: calories 148, fat 7.8, fiber 1.3, carbs 3.2, protein 16

Chicken with Almond Gravy

Prep time: 10 minutes | **Cook time:** 15 minutes | **Yield:** 2 servings

Ingredients

- 12 oz chicken breast, skinless, boneless
- ½ teaspoon salt
- ½ teaspoon white pepper
- ½ teaspoon ground black pepper
- ½ cup organic almond milk
- ½ teaspoon paprika

Method

1. Mix up together salt, white pepper, ground black pepper, and paprika.
2. Rub the chicken breast with the spice mixture generously.
3. After this, place the chicken breast in the instant pot bowl.
4. Add almond milk and close the lid.
5. Set the "Poultry" program and cook the chicken for 8 minutes. NPR -5 minutes.
6. Slice the chicken breast and sprinkle with the remaining gravy.

Nutritional info per serve: calories 112, fat 5, fiber 0.3, carbs 2.6, protein 36.5

Indian Style Chicken

Prep time: 5 minutes | **Cook time:** 4 minutes | **Yield:** 2 servings

Ingredients

- ¼ teaspoon cumin seeds
- ½ teaspoon turmeric
- 1 teaspoon ground paprika
- ¾ teaspoon chili paste
- ½ teaspoon ground coriander
- ½ cup of coconut milk
- 14 oz chicken breast, skinless, boneless
- 1 tablespoon coconut oil

Method

1. Blend together the cumin seeds, turmeric, ground paprika, chili paste, coriander, coconut milk, and coconut oil.
2. When the mixture is smooth – pour it in the instant pot bowl.
3. Chop the chicken breast roughly and transfer it in the spice mixture. Stir gently with the help of the spatula.
4. Lock the lid and seal it.
5. Set the "Manual" mode for 4 minutes (High pressure).
6. After this, make quick-release pressure.

Nutritional info per serve: calories 435, fat 26.6, fiber 1.9, carbs 5.1, protein 43.8

Mexican Bowl

Prep time: 8 minutes | **Cook time:** 12 minutes | **Yield:** 3 servings

Ingredients

- 10 oz chicken fillet
- 5 oz avocado, cored
- 1 teaspoon butter
- 1 tablespoon Mexican style seasonings
- 3 tablespoons coconut milk

Method

1. Cut the chicken fillet into the strips and sprinkle with the Mexican style seasonings.
2. Place the chicken in the instant pot bowl and add butter and coconut milk.
3. Set the "Poultry" program and cook it for 7 minutes (naturally release for 5 minutes).
4. Meanwhile, slice avocado and place it into the serving bowls.
5. Add the cooked chicken strips.

Nutritional info per serve: calories 329, fat 21.1, fiber 3.5, carbs 6.4, protein 28.6

White Mushrooms Poultry Stew

Prep time: 10 minutes | **Cook time:** 30 minutes | **Yield:** 2 servings

Ingredients

- 10 oz chicken breast, skinless, boneless
- 4 oz white mushrooms
- ¼ teaspoon salt
- ½ teaspoon white pepper
- ¾ teaspoon onion powder
- ½ teaspoon butter
- ¾ cup of water
- 1 tablespoon coconut cream

Method

1. Chop the chicken breast roughly and place it in the instant pot bowl.

2. Add salt, white pepper, onion powder, and water.

3. Set the "Saute" mode and start to cook the poultry.

4. Meanwhile, slice the mushrooms.

5. Add chopped white mushrooms in the instant pot bowl.

6. Add coconut cream and stir it.

7. Close the lid and seal it. Set the timer for 25 minutes.

   Nutritional info per serve: calories 204, fat 6.5, fiber 0.9, carbs 3.4, protein 32.2

Easy and Fast Chicken Drumsticks

Prep time: 10 minutes | **Cook time:** 10 minutes | **Yield:** 2 servings

Ingredients

- 4 chicken drumsticks
- 1 egg, whisked
- ½ teaspoon salt
- 1 tablespoon almond
- milk
- 1 tablespoon olive oil
- 1 cup water, for cooking

Method

1. In the mixing bowl mix up chicken drumsticks, salt, almond milk, and whisked egg.

2. Then massage the chicken with olive oil and transfer in the baking pan.

3. Pour water in the instant pot. Insert the baking pan with chicken.

4. Set the "Manual" mode and High pressure and cook the chicken for 10 minutes.

5. Make a quick pressure release and open the lid.

   Nutritional info per serve: calories 264, fat 16.2, fiber 0.2, carbs 0.6, protein 28.2

Marjoram Chicken Wings

Prep time: 7 minutes | **Cook time:** 10 minutes | **Yield:** 2 servings

Ingredients

- 1 teaspoon marjoram
- 1 teaspoon cream cheese
- ½ green pepper
- ½ teaspoon salt
- ½ teaspoon ground black pepper
- 14 oz chicken wings
- ¾ cup of water
- 1 teaspoon coconut oil

Method

1. Rub the chicken wings with the marjoram, salt, and ground black pepper.

2. Blend the green pepper until you get a puree.

3. Rub the chicken wings in the green pepper puree.

4. Then toss the coconut oil in the instant pot bowl and preheat it on the "Saute" mode.

5. Add the chicken wings and cook them for 3 minutes from each side or until light brown.

6. Then add cream cheese and water.

7. Cook the meal on "Manual" mode and put the timer for 4 minutes + High Pressure.

8. When the time is over – make a quick pressure release.

9. Let the cooked chicken wings chill for 1-2 minutes and serve them!

   Nutritional info per serve: calories 411, fat 17.7, fiber 0.8, carbs 1.9, protein 57.9

Chicken with Adobo Peppers

Prep time: 15 minutes | **Cook time:** 12 minutes | **Yield:** 2 servings

Ingredients

- 4 chicken thighs
- 2 tablespoons chipotle peppers in
- Adobo sauce
- ½ cup of water

Method

1. Pour water in the instant pot bowl.

2. Add chicken thighs and chipotle peppers in Adobo sauce.

3. Set the "Manual" mode (High pressure).

4. Turn on the timer for 12 minutes.

5. Make the natural pressure release for 10 minutes.

   Nutritional info per serve: calories 326, fat 20.5, fiber 1, carbs 0.5, protein 38.5

Bacon Chicken

Prep time: 15 minutes | **Cook time:** 15 minutes | **Yield:** 3 servings

Ingredients

- 12 oz chicken breast, boneless, skinless
- 5 oz bacon, sliced
- ½ teaspoon cayenne pepper
- ½ teaspoon ground white pepper
- ½ teaspoon minced garlic
- 1 teaspoon salt
- 1 tablespoon butter
- ¾ cup of water

Method

1. Stir together cayenne pepper, ground white pepper, minced garlic, and salt.
2. Then beat the chicken breast with the help of the kitchen hammer gently. It will make the final taste of meat tender and juicy.
3. Pu the butter and bacon on it.
4. Roll up the chicken breast to make the roll.
5. Secure the chicken roll with the help of the kitchen twine.
6. Wrap the roll into the foil.
7. Pour 1 cup of water in the instant pot bowl and place the trivet.
8. Place the chicken roll on the trivet and close the lid.
9. Set the "Steam" mode and High pressure.
10. Cook the chicken roll for 15 minutes. Then use the natural pressure release method.

Nutritional info per serve: calories 421, fat 26.5, fiber 0.2, carbs 1.2, protein 41.7

Green Sandwich

Prep time: 10 minutes | **Cook time:** 10 minutes | **Yield:** 2 servings

Ingredients

- 4 oz kale leaves
- 8 oz chicken fillet
- 1 tablespoon butter
- 1 oz lemon
- ¼ cup of water

Method

1. Dice the chicken fillet.
2. Squeeze the lemon juice over the poultry.
3. Transfer the poultry into the instant pot; add water and butter.
4. Close the lid and cook the chicken on the "Poultry" mode for 10 minutes.
5. When the chicken is cooked – place it on the kale leaves to make the medium sandwiches.

Nutritional info per serve: calories 298, fat 14.2, fiber 1.3, carbs.7.2, protein 34.7

Chicken Drumsticks de Provance

Prep time: 10 minutes | **Cook time:** 15 minutes | **Yield:** 2 servings

Ingredients

- 1 tablespoon herbs de Provance
- 4 chicken drumstick
- ¼ cup full-fat cream
- 1 teaspoon butter

Method

1. Rub the chicken drumstick with the herbs de Provance.
2. Melt the butter and mix it up with the full-fat cream.
3. Place the chicken drumstick on the foil and sprinkle with the creamy liquid.
4. Pour 1 cup of water in the instant pot and place the trivet there.
5. Transfer the chicken on the instant pot trivet.
6. Lock the instant pot lid and seal it.
7. Set the "Poultry" mode and timer for 15 minutes (High pressure).
8. When the poultry is cooked – use the quick pressure release method.

Nutritional info per serve: calories 192, fat 8.8, fiber 0, carbs 0.9, protein 25.6

Chicken Shish

Prep time: 10 minutes | **Cook time:** 5 minutes | **Yield:** 2 servings

Ingredients

- 1 tablespoon lemon juice
- ½ teaspoon cayenne pepper
- ½ teaspoon salt
- 10 oz chicken fillet
- 1 tablespoon avocado oil

Method

1. Chop the fillet into the medium cubes.
2. Sprinkle the chicken with the lemon juice, cayenne pepper, salt, and avocado oil.
3. Let it marinate for 10 minutes. After this, string the ingredients on the skewers.
4. Place them in the baking pan.
5. Pour 1 cup of water in the instant pot and place trivet.
6. Transfer the baking pan in the instant pot, on the trivet. Sprinkle the chicken with the remaining oil mixture.
7. Lock the instant pot lid and set "Manual" mode (High Pressure).
8. Set timer for 5 minutes. After this, make a quick pressure release.

Nutritional info per serve: calories 282, fat 11.5, fiber 0.5, carbs 0.8, protein 41.2

Pecorino Chicken Cubes

Prep time: 10 minutes | **Cook time:** 15 minutes | **Yield:** 3 servings

Ingredients

- 2 oz Pecorino cheese, grated
- 10 oz chicken breast, skinless, boneless
- 1 tablespoon butter
- ¾ cup heavy cream
- ½ teaspoon salt
- ½ teaspoon red hot pepper

Method

1. Chop the chicken breast into the cubes.

2. Toss butter in the instant pot and preheat it on the "Saute" mode.

3. Add the chicken cubes.

4. Sprinkle the poultry with the salt and red hot pepper.

5. Add cream and mix up together all the ingredients.

6. Close the lid of the instant pot and seal it.

7. Set "Poultry" mode and put a timer on 15 minutes.

8. When the time is over – let the chicken rest for 5 minutes more.

9. Transfer the meal on the plates and sprinkle with the grated cheese. The cheese shouldn't melt immediately.

Nutritional info per serve: calories 340, fat 24.9, fiber 0, carbs 0.9, protein 28.3

Tomato Chicken

Prep time: 10 minutes | **Cook time:** 35 minutes | **Yield:** 2 servings

Ingredients

- 2 chicken legs
- 2 tomatoes, chopped
- 1 cup chicken stock
- 1 teaspoon peppercorns

Method

1. Put all ingredients in the instant pot.

2. Close and seal the lid. Set "Manual" mode (high pressure).

3. Cook the chicken legs for 35 minutes.

4. Make a quick pressure release.

5. Transfer the cooked chicken legs in the serving bowls and add 1 ladle of the chicken stock.

Nutritional info per serve: calories 294, fat 15.9, fiber 1.8, carbs 5.8, protein 31.1

Herbed Chicken Balls

Prep time: 10 minutes | **Cook time:** 15 minutes | **Yield:** 2 servings

Ingredients

- 10 oz chicken fillet
- 1 egg
- 1 tablespoon almond flour
- ¾ teaspoon salt
- ¾ teaspoon paprika
- 1 teaspoon thyme
- ½ teaspoon butter
- ¾ teaspoon dried dill
- 1 cup water, for cooking

Method

1. Chop the chicken fillet into the tiny pieces.

2. Mix up together the almond flour, thyme, and dried dill. Stir the mixture gently.

3. After this, combine together the chicken and almond flour mixture. Stir it well and crack the egg in the mixture. Mix it up until smooth.

4. Make the medium balls from the mixture.

5. Grease the instant pot pan with the butter and place the balls.

6. Add 1 cup of water and close the instant pot.

7. Set the "Manual" program (High pressure) for 8 minutes.

8. After this, make quick release and chill the balls little.

Nutritional info per serve: calories 336, fat 15.5, fiber 0.9, carbs 2.1, protein 44.8

Mini Chicken Hashes

Prep time: 15 minutes | **Cook time:** 7 minutes | **Yield:** 2 servings

Ingredients

- 2 oz scallions, chopped
- ¾ cup of water
- 1 teaspoon coconut milk
- ½ teaspoon almond butter
- ½ teaspoon ground black pepper
- 10 oz chicken fillet, diced

Method

1. Set the "Stew" mode and toss the almond butter in the instant pot.

2. When the almond butter is melted – add the diced chicken.

3. Sprinkle it with the ground black pepper, chopped scallions, and add water.

4. Add coconut milk. Close the lid and cook the meal for 7 minutes (High pressure).

5. Make the natural pressure release for 10 minutes.

Nutritional info per serve: calories 310, fat 13.4, fiber 1.3, carbs 3.3, protein 42.5

Fish & Seafood

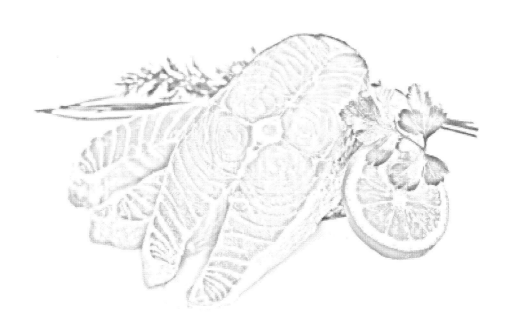

Bang Bang Shrimps

Prep time: 10 minutes | **Cook time:** 5 minutes | **Yield:** 4 servings

Ingredients

- 1-pound shrimps, peeled
- ½ cup almond flour
- 1 tablespoon olive oil
- ½ teaspoon salt
- 1 tablespoon mascarpone cheese

Method

1. In the mixing bowl, mix up salt and almond flour.
2. Then dip the shrimps in the mascarpone cheese and coat in the almond flour.
3. Heat up the olive oil in the instant pot on saute mode for 2 minutes.
4. Put the coated shrimps in the instant pot and cook them on saute mode for 1.5 minutes from each side.

   Nutritional info per serve: calories 256, fat 12.6, fiber 1.5, carbs .4.8, protein 29.3

Apple Cider Vinegar Mussels

Prep time: 10 minutes | **Cook time:** 5 minutes | **Yield:** 6 servings

Ingredients

- 18 oz mussels, fresh
- 1 cup apple cider vinegar
- 1 teaspoon coconut oil, melted
- ¼ cup of water
- 1 teaspoon minced garlic

Method

1. Pour water and apple cider vinegar in the instant pot.
2. Then insert the steamer rack.
3. Put the mussels in the instant pot mold.
4. Sprinkle them with coconut oil and minced garlic.
5. Close and seal the lid.
6. Cook the seafood on manual (high pressure) for 3 minutes. Make a quick pressure release.
7. If the mussels are not opened, cook them 2 minutes extra.

   Nutritional info per serve: calories 89, fat 2.7, fiber 0, carbs 3.7, protein 10.2

Thyme Lobster Tails

Prep time: 10 minutes | **Cook time:** 4 minutes | **Yield:** 4 servings

Ingredients

- 4 lobster tails
- 1 tablespoon butter, softened
- 1 teaspoon dried thyme
- 1 cup of water

Method

1. Pour water and insert the steamer rack in the instant pot.
2. Put the lobster tails on the rack and close the lid.
3. Cook the meal on manual mode (high pressure) for 4 minutes. Make a quick pressure release.
4. After this, mix up butter and dried thyme.
5. Peel the lobsters and rub them with thyme butter.

   Nutritional info per serve: calories 126, fat 2.9, fiber 0.1, carbs 0.2, protein 24.1

Blackened Salmon

Prep time: 10 minutes | **Cook time:** 4 minutes | **Yield:** 3 servings

Ingredients

- 1-pound salmon fillet
- 1 teaspoon ground black pepper
- ½ teaspoon salt
- 1 teaspoon ground turmeric
- 1 teaspoon lemon juice
- 1 cup of water

Method

1. In the shallow bowl, mix up salt, ground black pepper, and ground turmeric.
2. Sprinkle the salmon fillet with lemon juice and rub with the spice mixture.
3. Then pour water in the instant pot and insert the steamer rack.
4. Wrap the salmon fillet in the foil and place it on the rack.
5. Close and seal the lid.
6. Cook the fish on manual mode (high pressure) for 4 minutes.
7. Make a quick pressure release and cut the fish on servings.

   Nutritional info per serve: calories 205, fat 9.4, fiber 0.4, carbs 1, protein 29.5

Shrimp Curry with Coconut Milk

Prep time: 10 minutes | **Cook time:** 4 minutes | **Yield:** 5 servings

Ingredients

- 15 oz shrimps, peeled
- 1 teaspoon chili powder
- 1 teaspoon garam masala
- 1 cup of coconut milk
- 1 teaspoon olive oil
- ½ teaspoon minced garlic

Method

1. Heat up the instant pot on saute mode for 2 minutes.
2. Then add olive oil. Cook the ingredients for 1 minute.
3. Add shrimps and sprinkle them with chili powder, garam masala, minced garlic, and coconut milk.
4. Carefully stir the ingredients and close the lid.
5. Cook the shrimp curry on manual mode for 1 minute. Make a quick pressure release.

Nutritional info per serve: calories 222, fat 13.9, fiber 1.3, carbs 4.4, protein 20.6

Chili Haddock

Prep time: 10 minutes | **Cook time:** 5 minutes | **Yield:** 4 servings

Ingredients

- 1 chili pepper, minced
- 1-pound haddock, chopped
- ½ teaspoon ground turmeric
- ½ cup fish stock
- 1 cup of water

Method

1. In the mixing bowl mix up chili pepper, ground turmeric, and fish stock.
2. Then add chopped haddock and transfer the mixture in the baking mold.
3. Pour water in the instant pot and insert the trivet.
4. Place the baking mold with fish on the trivet and close the lid.
5. Cook the meal on manual (high pressure) for 5 minutes. Make a quick pressure release.

Nutritional info per serve: calories 130, fat 1.1, fiber 0.1, carbs 0.3, protein 28

Spinach Tuna Cakes

Prep time: 15 minutes | **Cook time:** 8 minutes | **Yield:** 4 servings

Ingredients

- 10 oz tuna, grinded
- 1 cup spinach
- 1 egg, beaten
- 1 teaspoon ground coriander
- 2 tablespoon coconut flakes
- 1 tablespoon avocado oil

Method

1. Blend the spinach in the blender until smooth.
2. Then transfer it in the mixing bowl and add grinded tuna, egg, and ground coriander.
3. Add coconut flakes and stir the mass with the help of the spoon.
4. Heat up avocado oil in the instant pot on saute mode for 2 minutes.
5. Then make the medium size cakes from the tuna mixture and place them in the hot oil.
6. Cook the tuna cakes on saute mode for 3 minutes.
7. Then flip the on another side and cook for 3 minutes more or until they are light brown.

Nutritional info per serve: calories 163, fat 8.1, fiber 0.6, carbs 0.9, protein 20.5

Seafood Zoodle Alfredo

Prep time: 10 minutes | **Cook time:** 10 minutes | **Yield:** 4 servings

Ingredients

- 2 zucchinis, trimmed
- 1 cup coconut cream
- 1 teaspoon butter
- 1 teaspoon seafood seasonings
- 6 oz shrimps, peeled

Method

1. Melt the butter on saute mode and add shrimps.
2. Sprinkle them with seafood seasonings and saute then for 2 minutes.
3. After this, spiralizer the zucchini with the help of the spiralizer and add in the shrimps.
4. Add coconut cream and close the lid. Cook the meal on saute mode for 8 minutes.

Nutritional info per serve: calories 213, fat 16.2, fiber 2.4, carbs 7.3, protein 12.3

Lemon Salmon

Prep time: 10 minutes | **Cook time:** 4 minutes | **Yield:** 4 servings

Ingredients

- 1-pound salmon fillet
- 1 tablespoon butter, melted
- 2 tablespoons lemon
- juice
- 1 teaspoon dried dill
- 1 cup of water

Method

1. Cut the salmon fillet on 4 servings.

2. Line the instant pot baking pan with foil and put the salmon fillets inside in one layer.

3. Then sprinkle the fish with dried dill, lemon juice, and butter.

4. Pour water in the instant pot and insert the rack.

5. Place the baking pan with salmon on the rack and close the lid.

6. Cook the meal on manual mode (high pressure) for 4 minutes. Allow the natural pressure release for 5 minutes and remove the fish from the instant pot.

Nutritional info per serve: calories 178, fat 10, fiber 0.1, carbs 0.3, protein 22.1

Alaskan Crab Legs

Prep time: 10 minutes | **Cook time:** 4 minutes | **Yield:** 4 servings

Ingredients

- 1-pound Alaskan crab legs
- 1 tablespoon butter
- ¼ teaspoon dried cilantro
- 1 cup of water

Method

1. Pour water in the instant pot.

2. Add dried cilantro and crab legs.

3. Cook the on manual mode (high pressure) for 4 minutes.

4. Then make a quick pressure release.

5. Peel the crab legs and sprinkle them with butter.

Nutritional info per serve: calories 78, fat 3.3, fiber 0.1, carbs 0.3, protein 12

Cajun Cod

Prep time: 10 minutes | **Cook time:** 4 minutes | **Yield:** 2 servings

Ingredients

- 10 oz cod fillet
- 1 tablespoon olive oil
- 1 teaspoon Cajun
- seasonings
- 2 tablespoons coconut aminos

Method

1. Sprinkle the cod fillet with coconut aminos and Cajun seasonings.

2. Then heat up olive oil in the instant pot on saute mode.

3. Add the spiced cod fillet and cook it for 4 minutes from each side.

4. Then cut it into halves and sprinkle with the oily liquid from the instant pot.

Nutritional info per serve: calories 189, fat 8.3, fiber 0, carbs 3, protein 25.3

Salmon Caprese

Prep time: 10 minutes | **Cook time:** 15 minutes | **Yield:** 2 servings

Ingredients

- 10 oz salmon fillet (2 fillets)
- 4 oz Mozzarella, sliced
- 4 cherry tomatoes, sliced
- 1 teaspoon Erythritol
- 1 teaspoon dried
- basil
- ½ teaspoon ground black pepper
- 1 tablespoon apple cider vinegar
- 1 tablespoon butter
- 1 cup water, for cooking

Method

1. Grease the mold with butter and put the salmon inside.

2. Sprinkle the fish with Erythritol, dried basil, ground black pepper, and apple cider vinegar.

3. Then top the salmon with tomatoes and Mozzarella.

4. Pour water and insert the steamer rack in the instant pot.

5. Put the fish on the rack.

6. Close and seal the lid.

7. Cook the meal on manual mode (high pressure0 for 15 minutes. Make a quick pressure release.

Nutritional info per serve: calories 447, fat 25, fiber 3.2, carbs 14.8, protein 45.9

Clam Chowder

Prep time: 10 minutes | **Cook time:** 4 minutes | **Yield:** 2 servings

Ingredients

- 5 oz clams
- 1 oz bacon, chopped
- 3 oz celery, chopped
- ½ cup of water
- ½ cup heavy cream

Method

1. Cook the bacon on saute mode for 1 minute.
2. Then add clams, celery, water, and heavy cream.
3. Close and seal the lid.
4. Cook the seafood on steam mode (high pressure) for 3 minutes. Make a quick pressure release.
5. Ladle the clams with the heavy cream mixture in the bowls.

Nutritional info per serve: calories 221, fat 17.2, fiber 1, carbs 10.1, protein 6.6

Rosemary Catfish Steak

Prep time: 10 minutes | **Cook time:** 20 minutes | **Yield:** 4 servings

Ingredients

- 16 oz catfish fillet
- 1 tablespoon dried rosemary
- 1 teaspoon garlic powder
- 1 tablespoon avocado oil
- 1 teaspoon salt
- 1 cup water, for cooking

Method

1. Cut the catfish fillet into 4 steaks.
2. Then sprinkle them with dried rosemary, garlic powder, avocado oil, and salt.
3. Place the fish steak in the baking mold in one layer.
4. After this, pour water and insert the steamer rack in the instant pot.
5. Put the baking mold with fish on the rack. Close and seal the lid.
6. Cook the meal on manual (high pressure) for 20 minutes. Make a quick pressure release.

Nutritional info per serve: calories 163, fat 9.2, fiber 0.6, carbs 1.2, protein 17.8

Louisiana Gumbo

Prep time: 10 minutes | **Cook time:** 4 minutes | **Yield:** 6 servings

Ingredients

- 1-pound shrimps
- ¼ cup celery stalk, chopped
- 1 chili pepper, chopped
- ¼ cup okra, chopped
- 1 tablespoon coconut oil
- 2 cups chicken broth
- 1 teaspoon tomato paste

Method

1. Put all ingredients in the instant pot and stir until you get a light red color.
2. Then close and seal the lid.
3. Cook the meal on manual mode (high pressure) for 4 minutes.
4. When the time is finished, allow the natural pressure release for 10 minutes.

Nutritional info per serve: calories 126, fat 4, fiber 0.3, carbs 2.1, protein 19

Shrimp Skewers

Prep time: 10 minutes | **Cook time:** 2 minutes | **Yield:** 4 servings

Ingredients

- 1 tablespoon lemon juice
- 1 teaspoon coconut aminos
- 12 oz shrimps, peeled
- 1 teaspoon olive oil
- 1 cup of water

Method

1. Put the shrimps in the mixing bowl.
2. Add lemon juice, coconut aminos, and olive oil.
3. Then string the shrimps on the skewers.
4. Pour water in the instant pot.
5. Then insert the trivet.
6. Put the shrimp skewers on the trivet.
7. Close the lid and cook the seafood on manual mode (high pressure) for 2 minutes.
8. When the time is finished, make a quick pressure release.

Nutritional info per serve: calories 113, fat 2.6, fiber 0, carbs 1.6, protein 19.4

Butter Clams

Prep time: 10 minutes | **Cook time:** 3 minutes | **Yield:** 2 servings

Ingredients

- 7 oz clams
- 2 tablespoons butter
- 1 cup of water
- 1 teaspoon minced garlic

Method

1. Pour water in the instant pot.
2. Add clams and close the lid.
3. Cook the cams on high pressure for 3 minutes.
4. When the time is over, make a quick pressure release and transfer the hot clams in the bowl.
5. Add butter and minced garlic.
6. Shake the seafood well.

Nutritional info per serve: calories 152, fat 11.7, fiber 0.4, carbs 11.3, protein 0.8

Lime Mahi Mahi

Prep time: 10 minutes | **Cook time:** 9 minutes | **Yield:** 4 servings

Ingredients

- 1-pound mahi-mahi fillet
- 1 teaspoon lemon zest, grated
- 1 tablespoon lemon juice
- 1 tablespoon butter, softened
- ½ teaspoon salt
- 1 cup water, for cooking

Method

1. Cut the fish on 4 servings and sprinkle with lemon zest, lemon juice, salt, and rub with softened butter.
2. Then put the fish in the baking pan in one layer.
3. Pour water and insert the steamer rack in the instant pot.
4. Put the mold with fish on the rack. Close and seal the lid.
5. Cook the Mahi Mahi on manual mode (high pressure) for 9 minutes. Make a quick pressure release.

Nutritional info per serve: calories 128, fat 4, fiber 0.1, carbs 0.2, protein 21.5

Salmon Pate

Prep time: 10 minutes | **Cook time:** 15 minutes | **Yield:** 6 servings

Ingredients

- 1-pound salmon
- 2 tablespoons cream cheese
- ½ teaspoon salt
- 1 teaspoon chives, chopped
- 1 cup water, for cooking

Method

1. Put salmon and water in the instant pot.
2. Close and seal the lid and cook the fish on manual (high pressure) mode for 15 minutes.
3. Make a quick pressure release and transfer the salmon in the food processor.
4. Add salt, chives, and cream cheese. Blend the fish mixture until smooth.
5. Transfer the cooked pate in the glass jar.

Nutritional info per serve: calories 112, fat 5.8, fiber 0, carbs 0.1, protein 14.9

Mackerel Casserole

Prep time: 15 minutes | **Cook time:** 15 minutes | **Yield:** 5 servings

Ingredients

- 1 cup broccoli, shredded
- 10 oz mackerel, chopped
- ½ cup Cheddar
- cheese, shredded
- 1 cup of coconut milk
- 1 teaspoon ground cumin
- 1 teaspoon salt

Method

1. Sprinkle the chopped mackerel with ground cumin and salt and transfer in the instant pot.
2. Top the fish with shredded broccoli and Cheddar cheese,
3. Then add coconut milk. Close and seal the lid.
4. Cook the casserole on manual mode (high pressure) for 15 minutes.
5. Allow the natural pressure release for 10 minutes and open the lid.

Nutritional info per serve: calories 312, fat 25.4, fiber 1.6, carbs 4.2, protein 18

Spicy Cod

Prep time: 10 minutes | **Cook time:** 10 minutes | **Yield:** 2 servings

Ingredients

- 2 cod fillet
- ¼ teaspoon chili powder
- ½ teaspoon cayenne pepper
- ½ teaspoon dried oregano
- 1 tablespoon lime juice
- 2 tablespoons avocado oil

Method

1. Rub the cod fillets with chili powder, cayenne pepper, dried oregano, and sprinkle with lime juice.

2. Then pour the avocado oil in the instant pot and heat it up on saute mode for 2 minutes.

3. Put the cod fillets in the hot oil and cook for 5 minutes.

4. Then flip the fish on another side and cook for 5 minutes more.

Nutritional info per serve: calories 114, fat 3, fiber 1, carbs 2, protein 20.3

Pulpo Gallego

Prep time: 10 minutes | **Cook time:** 15 minutes | **Yield:** 4 servings

Ingredients

- 1-pound octopus, rinsed
- 1 garlic clove, diced
- 1 teaspoon salt
- 1 tablespoon avocado oil
- 1 cup of water

Method

1. Put the octopus in the instant pot.

2. Add avocado oil, salt, and diced garlic. Mix up the ingredients and add water.

3. Close and seal the lid.

4. Cook the meal on manual mode (high pressure) for 15 minutes.

5. Then allow the natural pressure release for 10 minutes.

6. Transfer the cooked octopus on the serving plate.

Nutritional info per serve: calories 192, fat 2.8, fiber 0.2, carbs 5.4, protein 33.9

Cod Lime Pieces

Prep time: 10 minutes | **Cook time:** 9 minutes | **Yield:** 2 servings

Ingredients

- 6 oz cod fillet
- 1 teaspoon lime zest, grated
- 1 tablespoon lime juice
- 1 tablespoon coconut oil
- 1 egg, beaten

Method

1. Cut the cod fillet into medium cubes and sprinkle with lime juice and lime zest.

2. Then dip the fish cubes in the egg.

3. Heat up coconut oil on saute mode for 3 minutes.

4. Put the cod cubes in the hot oil in one layer and cook on saute mode for 4 minutes.

5. Then flip the on another side and cook for 2 minutes more.

Nutritional info per serve: calories 161, fat 9.8, fiber 0.1, carbs 0.9, protein 18

Crustless Fish Pie

Prep time: 15 minutes | **Cook time:** 15 minutes | **Yield:** 6 servings

Ingredients

- 1 cup cauliflower, boiled, mashed
- 3 eggs, hard-boiled, peeled, chopped
- 10 oz salmon, chopped, boiled
- ½ cup mozzarella cheese, shredded
- ½ cup heavy cream
- ¼ cup chicken broth
- 1 teaspoon salt
- ½ teaspoon ground paprika

Method

1. Mix up chopped salmon and eggs and transfer them in the instant pot bowl.

2. Sprinkle the mixture with salt and ground paprika.

3. After this, top it with mashed cauliflower and mozzarella.

4. Add chicken broth and heavy cream.

5. Close and seal the lid.

6. Cook the pie for 15 minutes on manual mode (high pressure). Make a quick pressure release.

Nutritional info per serve: calories 141, fat 9.3, fiber 0.5, carbs 1.6, protein 13.4

Flounder Meuniere

Prep time: 15 minutes | **Cook time:** 10 minutes | **Yield:** 4 servings

Ingredients

- 16 oz flounder fillet
- ½ teaspoon ground black pepper
- ½ teaspoon salt
- ½ cup almond flour
- 2 tablespoons olive oil
- 1 tablespoon lemon juice
- 1 teaspoon fresh parsley, chopped

Method

1. Cut the fish fillets into 4 servings and sprinkle with salt, ground black pepper, and lemon juice.
2. Heat up the instant pot on saute mode for 2 minutes and add olive oil.
3. Coat the flounder fillets in the almond flour and put them in the hot olive oil.
4. Saute the fish fillets for 4 minutes and then flip on another side.
5. Cook the meal for 3 minutes more or until it is golden brown.
6. Sprinkle the cooked flounder with the fresh parsley.

Nutritional info per serve: calories 214, fat 10.5, fiber 0.5, carbs 1, protein 28.2

Salmon Loaf

Prep time: 15 minutes | **Cook time:** 25 minutes | **Yield:** 6 servings

Ingredients

- 12 oz salmon, boiled, shredded
- 3 eggs, beaten
- ½ cup almond flour
- 1 teaspoon garlic powder
- ¼ cup parmesan, grated
- 1 teaspoon butter, softened
- 1 cup water, for cooking

Method

1. Pour water in the instant pot.
2. Mix up the rest of the ingredients in the mixing bowl and stir until smooth.
3. After this, transfer the salmon mixture in the loaf pan and flatten; insert the pan in the instant pot. Close and seal the lid.
4. Cook the meal on manual mode (high pressure) for 25 minutes.
5. When the cooking time is finished, make a quick pressure release and cool the loaf well before serving.

Nutritional info per serve: calories 172, fat 10.5, fiber 0.3, carbs 1.5, protein 18.9

Lemon Halibut

Prep time: 10 minutes | **Cook time:** 9 minutes | **Yield:** 3 servings

Ingredients

- 3 halibut fillet
- ½ lemon, sliced
- ½ teaspoon white pepper
- ½ teaspoon ground
- coriander
- 1 tablespoon avocado oil
- 1 cup water, for cooking

Method

1. Pour water and insert the steamer rack in the instant pot.
2. Rub the fish fillets with white pepper, ground coriander, and avocado oil.
3. Place the fillets in the steamer rack.
4. Then top the halibut with sliced lemon. Close and seal the lid.
5. Cook the meal on High pressure for 9 minutes. Make a quick pressure release.

Nutritional info per serve: calories 328, fat 7.3, fiber 0.6, carbs 1.4, protein 60.7

Mozzarella Fish Sticks

Prep time: 15 minutes | **Cook time:** 7 minutes | **Yield:** 6 servings

Ingredients

- 10 oz cod fillet, grinded
- 1 egg, beaten
- 2 tablespoons flax meal
- ¼ cup Mozzarella, shredded
- 1 tablespoon coconut flakes
- 1/3 cup coconut oil

Method

1. In the mixing bowl, mix up grinded cod fillet, egg, and shredded Mozzarella.
2. Then mix up flax meal and coconut flakes.
3. After this, make the small sticks from the cheese mixture and coat them in the coconut flakes mixture.
4. Bring the coconut oil to boil on saute mode.
5. Put the fish sticks in the hot coconut oil and saute them for 2 minutes or until the sticks are light brown.
6. Dry the cooked mozzarella fish sticks with the paper towel.

Nutritional info per serve: calories 169, fat 14.6, fiber 0.7, carbs 0.9, protein 10.2

Fish Cream Cheese Casserole

Prep time: 7 minutes | **Cook time:** 5 minutes | **Yield:** 2 servings

Ingredients

- 1 teaspoon chili flakes
- 10 oz tuna, chopped
- ½ teaspoon salt
- 2 tablespoons cream cheese
- 1 teaspoon coconut oil

Method

1. Take the springform pan and grease it with the coconut oil.
2. Make the layer of tuna in the springform pan.
3. After this, put the layer of the cream cheese.
4. Sprinkle the casserole with the salt and chili flakes.
5. Top the casserole with the cream cheese.
6. Pour 1 cup of water in the instant pot bowl and place the trivet.
7. Put the casserole on the trivet and wrap it with the foil.
8. Set "Manual" mode (High pressure) for 5 minutes -QPR.
9. Chill the casserole little.

Nutritional info per serve: calories 318, fat 17.2, fiber 0, carbs 0.3, protein 38.4

Italian Style Salmon

Prep time: 10 minutes | **Cook time:** 4 minutes | **Yield:** 2 servings

Ingredients

- 10 oz salmon fillet
- 1 teaspoon Italian
- seasonings
- 1 cup of water

Method

1. Pour water and insert the trivet in the instant pot.
2. Then rub the salmon fillet with Italian seasonings and wrap in the foil.
3. Place the wrapped fish on the trivet and close the lid.
4. Cook the meal on manual mode (high pressure) for 4 minutes.
5. Make a quick pressure release and remove the fish from the foil.
6. Cut it into servings.

Nutritional info per serve: calories 195, fat 9.5, fiber 0, carbs 0.3, protein 27.5

Lobster Cakes

Prep time: 10 minutes | **Cook time:** 10 minutes | **Yield:** 6 servings

Ingredients

- 1-pound lobster meat, grinded
- 1 egg, beaten
- 2 oz scallions, chopped
- ¼ cup coconut flour
- ½ teaspoon chili flakes
- 3 tablespoons coconut oil

Method

1. Heat up coconut oil for 2 minutes on saute mode.
2. Meanwhile, mix up lobster meat, egg, scallions, coconut flour, and chili flakes. Make the medium size cakes and put them in the hot coconut oil.
3. Saute the lobster cakes for 5 minutes per side or until they are golden brown.

Nutritional info per serve: calories 160, fat 9.4, fiber 2.3, carbs 5.5, protein 11.2

Flounder Baked with Artichokes

Prep time: 10 minutes | **Cook time:** 10 minutes | **Yield:** 2 servings

Ingredients

- 8 oz flounder fillet
- 1 lemon slice, chopped
- 1 teaspoon ground black pepper
- ¼ teaspoon salt
- ½ large artichoke, chopped
- 1 tablespoon sesame oil
- 1 cup water, for cooking

Method

1. Brush the round baking pan with sesame oil.
2. Then place the chopped artichoke in the baking pan and flatten it.
3. Sprinkle the flounder fillet with ground black pepper and salt and put over the artichoke.
4. Add chopped lemon.
5. Pour water and insert the steamer rack in the instant pot.
6. Place the pan with fish in the steamer. Close and seal the lid.
7. Cook the meal on manual (high pressure) for 10 minutes. Make a quick pressure release.

Nutritional info per serve: calories 216, fat 8.6, fiber 2.6, carbs 5.3, protein 28.9

Cod with Olives

Prep time: 15 minutes | **Cook time:** 10 minutes | **Yield:** 2 servings

Ingredients

- 8 oz cod fillet
- ¼ cup olives, sliced
- 1 teaspoon olive oil
- ¼ teaspoon salt
- 1 cup water, for cooking

Method

1. Pour water and insert the steamer rack in the instant pot.
2. Then cut the cod fillet into 2 servings and sprinkle with salt and olive oil.
3. Then place the fish on the foil and top with the sliced olives. Wrap the fish and transfer it in the steamer rack.
4. Close and seal the lid. Cook the fish on manual mode (high pressure) for 10 minutes.
5. Allow the natural pressure release for 5 minutes.

Nutritional info per serve: calories 130, fat 5.1, fiber 0.5, carbs 1.1, protein 20.4

Haddock under Spinach Blanket

Prep time: 15 minutes | **Cook time:** 15 minutes | **Yield:** 4 servings

Ingredients

- 12 oz haddock fillet
- 1 cup spinach
- 1 tablespoon avocado oil
- 1 teaspoon minced garlic
- ½ teaspoon ground coriander
- 1 cup water, for cooking

Method

1. Blend the spinach until smooth and mix up with avocado oil, ground coriander, and minced garlic.
2. Then cut the haddock into 4 fillets and place on the foil.
3. Top the fish fillets with spinach mixture and place them on the rack.
4. Pour water and insert the rack in the instant pot.
5. Close and seal the lid and cook the haddock on manual (high pressure) for 15 minutes.
6. Do the quick pressure release.

Nutritional info per serve: calories 103, fat 1.3, fiber 0.3, carbs 0.7, protein 20.9

Shrimp Ragout

Prep time: 5 minutes | **Cook time:** 8 minutes | **Yield:** 2 servings

Ingredients

- ½ cup of water
- ½ green pepper, chopped
- 1 teaspoon scallions, chopped
- 1 teaspoon turmeric
- ½ teaspoon salt
- 7 oz shrimps, peeled
- ¼ cup cauliflower, chopped

Method

1. Set "Saute" mode at instant pot.
2. When the "Hot" is displayed – pour water and inside.
3. Add all remaining ingredients.
4. Close the lid and change the "Saute" mode into "Manual" (High pressure).
5. Set the timer for 5 minutes.
6. When the time is over – use the quick pressure release method.

Nutritional info per serve: calories 131, fat 1.9, fiber 1.1, carbs 4.3, protein 23.2

Tender Salmon Fillets

Prep time: 10 minutes | **Cook time:** 10 minutes | **Yield:** 2 servings

Ingredients

- 1 tablespoon dried dill
- 10 oz salmon fillet (cut into 2 servings)
- ½ teaspoon salt
- 1 tablespoon cream cheese
- 1 tablespoon butter

Method

1. Gently rub the fish fillets with dill and salt.
2. Preheat the instant pot on the "Saute" mode until it is displayed "Hot".
3. Toss the butter inside and melt it.
4. Transfer the salmon fillets in the instant pot and cook them for 2 minutes from each side.
5. Add the cream cheese and saute the fish for 4 minutes more.

Nutritional info per serve: calories 260, fat 16.3, fiber 0.2, carbs 1, protein 28.3

Salmon Cakes

Prep time: 15 minutes | **Cook time:** 10 minutes | **Yield:** 4 servings

Ingredients

- 1-pound salmon fillet, chopped
- 1 tablespoon dill, chopped
- 2 eggs, beaten
- ½ cup almond flour
- 1 tablespoon coconut oil

Method

1. Put the chopped salmon, dill, eggs, and almond flour in the food processor.
2. Blend the mixture until it is smooth.
3. Then make the small balls (cakes) from the salmon mixture.
4. After this, heat up the coconut oil on saute mode for 3 minutes.
5. Put the salmon cakes in the instant pot in one layer and cook them on saute mode for 2 minutes from each side or until they are light brown.

Nutritional info per serve: calories 297, fat 19.3, fiber 1.6, carbs 3.6, protein 27.9

Pesto Flounder

Prep time: 15 minutes | **Cook time:** 15 minutes | **Yield:** 3 servings

Ingredients

- 2 tablespoons pesto sauce
- ½ cup butter
- 10 oz flounder fillet
- 1 cup water, for cooking

Method

1. Cut the fish into 3 servings and put in the baking pan.
2. Brush the flounder fillets with pesto sauce. Add butter.
3. Pour water and insert the steamer rack in the instant pot.
4. Put the baking pan with fish on the rack. Close and seal the lid.
5. Cook the meal on manual mode (high pressure) for 15 minutes. Allow the natural pressure release for 10 minutes.

Nutritional info per serve: calories 427, fat 36.5, fiber 0.2, carbs 0.7, protein 24.2

Butter Scallops

Prep time: 10 minutes | **Cook time:** 10 minutes | **Yield:** 4 servings

Ingredients

- 1-pound sea scallops
- 1 tablespoon coconut aminos
- ¼ cup apple cider vinegar
- 1 garlic clove, diced
- 1 teaspoon chili flakes
- ¼ teaspoon salt
- ¼ cup butter
- ½ cup beef broth

Method

1. Melt the butter on saute mode and add scallops.
2. Cook them for 2 minutes per side.
3. Add all remaining ingredients. Close and seal the lid.
4. Cook the scallops on manual mode (high pressure) for 3 minutes. Allow the natural pressure release for 5 minutes.

Nutritional info per serve: calories 214, fat 12.5, fiber 0, carbs 4, protein 19.8

Fish Nuggets

Prep time: 15 minutes | **Cook time:** 9 minutes | **Yield:** 4 servings

Ingredients

- 1-pound tilapia fillet
- ½ cup almond flour
- 3 eggs, beaten
- ¼ cup avocado oil
- 1 teaspoon salt

Method

1. Cut the fish into the small pieces (nuggets) and sprinkle withs alt.
2. Then dip the fish nuggets in the eggs and coat in the almond flour.
3. Heat up avocado oil for 3 minutes on saute mode.
4. Put the prepared fish nuggets in the hot oil and cook them on saute mode for 3 minutes from each side or until they are golden brown.

Nutritional info per serve: calories 179, fat 7.8, fiber 1, carbs 1.8, protein 26.2

Mascarpone Tilapia

Prep time: 10 minutes | **Cook time:** 20 minutes | **Yield:** 2 servings

Ingredients

- 10 oz tilapia
- ½ cup mascarpone
- 1 garlic clove, diced
- 1 teaspoon ground nutmeg
- 1 tablespoon olive oil
- ½ teaspoon salt

Method

1. Pour olive oil in the instant pot.
2. Add diced garlic and saute it for 4 minutes.
3. Add tilapia and sprinkle it with ground nutmeg. Saute the fish for 3 minutes per side.
4. Add mascarpone and close the lid.
5. Saute tilapia for 10 minutes.

   Nutritional info per serve: calories 293, fat 16.7, fiber 0.3, carbs 2.9, protein 33.5

Tuna Stuffed Poblanos

Prep time: 15 minutes | **Cook time:** 12 minutes | **Yield:** 4 servings

Ingredients

- 7 oz tuna, canned, shredded
- 1 teaspoon cream cheese
- ¼ teaspoon minced garlic
- 2 oz Provolone cheese, grated
- 4 poblano pepper
- 1 cup water, for cooking

Method

1. Remove the seeds from poblano peppers.
2. In the mixing bowl, mix up shredded tuna, cream cheese, minced garlic, and grated cheese.
3. Then fill the peppers with tuna mixture and put it in the baking pan.
4. Pour water and insert the baking pan in the instant pot.
5. Cook the meal on manual mode (high pressure) for 12 minutes. Then make a quick pressure release.

   Nutritional info per serve: calories 153, fat 8.1, fiber 1.3, carbs 2.2, protein 17.3

Sour Seabass

Prep time: 5 minutes | **Cook time:** 3 minutes | **Yield:** 2 servings

Ingredients

- 14 oz seabass steak
- 1 tablespoon lemon juice
- 1 tablespoon apple cider vinegar
- ¾ teaspoon salt
- ¾ cup of coconut milk
- ½ teaspoon minced garlic
- ½ teaspoon smoked paprika

Method

1. Mix up together the lemon juice, apple cider vinegar, salt, minced garlic, and smoked paprika.
2. Rub the seabass steak with the spice mixture and place it in the instant pot bowl.
3. Add coconut milk and lock the instant pot lid.
4. Set the "Manual" mode for 3 minutes. Make the quick-release pressure then.

   Nutritional info per serve: calories 619, fat 45.9, fiber 3.8, carbs 5.8, protein 47.3

Salmon with Dill

Prep time: 7 minutes | **Cook time:** 8 minutes | **Yield:** 2 servings

Ingredients

- 1 teaspoon salt
- 2 tablespoons fresh dill, chopped
- 10 oz salmon fillet
- ¼ cup butter
- ½ cup of water

Method

1. Put butter and salt in the baking pan.
2. Add salmon fillet and dill. Cover the pan with foil.
3. Pour water in the instant pot and insert the baking pan with fish inside.
4. Set the "Steam" mode and cook the salmon for 8 minutes.
5. Unwrap the cooked salmon and serve!

   Nutritional info per serve: calories 399, fat 31.9, fiber 0.4, carbs 1.8, protein 28.4

Haddock Bake

Prep time: 7 minutes | **Cook time:** 10 minutes | **Yield:** 2 servings

Ingredients

- 2 eggs, beaten
- 12 oz haddock fillet, chopped
- 1 tablespoon cream cheese
- ¾ teaspoon dried rosemary
- 2 oz Parmesan, grated
- 1 teaspoon butter

Method

1. Whisk the beaten eggs until homogenous. Add the cream cheese, dried rosemary, and dill.

2. Grease the springform with the butter and place the haddock inside.

3. Pour the egg mixture over the fish and add sprinkle with parmesan.

4. Set the "Manual" mode (High pressure) and cook for 5 minutes. Then make natural-release pressure for 5 minutes.

Nutritional info per serve: calories 380, fat 15.7, fiber 0.2, carbs 18, protein 56.3

Steamed Seabass

Prep time: 5 minutes | **Cook time:** 8 minutes | **Yield:** 2 servings

Ingredients

- 10 oz seabass steak
- 1 teaspoon salt
- 1 teaspoon ground
- black pepper
- 1 cup water, for cooking

Method

1. Rub the seabass steak with salt and ground black pepper.

2. Pour water and insert the steamer rack in the instant pot.

3. Place the fish on the rack. Close and seal the lid.

4. Cook the fish on the "Steam" mode for 8 minutes (Quick pressure release).

Nutritional info per serve: calories 292, fat 17.4, fiber 1.4, carbs 0.7, protein 32.3

Fish Curry

Prep time: 10 minutes | **Cook time:** 3 minutes | **Yield:** 2 servings

Ingredients

- 8 oz cod fillet, chopped
- 1 teaspoon curry
- paste
- 1 cup organic almond milk

Method

1. Mix up curry paste and almond milk and pour the liquid in the instant pot.

2. Add chopped cod fillet and close the lid.

3. Cook the fish curry on manual mode (high pressure) for 3 minutes. Then make the quick pressure release for 5 minutes.

Nutritional info per serve: calories 138, fat 3.7, fiber 0, carbs 4.7, protein 20.9

Spicy Fish Balls

Prep time: 8 minutes | **Cook time:** 10 minutes | **Yield:** 3 servings

Ingredients

- 1 tablespoon butter
- 15 oz cod
- ¼ teaspoon dried oregano
- 1 teaspoon ground nutmeg
- ½ teaspoon dried dill

Method

1. Grind the cod and mix it up with all spices.

2. Heat up the butter on saute mode.

3. Make the small balls from the cod mixture and put them in the hot butter.

4. Cook the fish balls for 3 minutes from each side on saute mode.

Nutritional info per serve: calories 187, fat 5.4, fiber 0.2, carbs 0.5, protein 32.5

Boiled Crawfish

Prep time: 5 minutes | **Cook time:** 5 minutes | **Yield:** 4 servings

Ingredients

- 16 oz crawfish
- 1 teaspoon old bay
- seasonings
- 1 cup of water

Method

1. Pour water in the instant pot bowl.

2. Add old bay seasonings and crawfish.

3. Close and seal the lid and cook the seafood on manual mode (high pressure) for 5 minutes.

4. Then make a quick pressure release and transfer the cooked crawfish in the plate.

Nutritional info per serve: calories 99, fat 1.5, fiber 0, carbs 0, protein 19.9

Coconut Squid

Prep time: 10 minutes | **Cook time:** 20 minutes | **Yield:** 3 servings

Ingredients

- 1-pound squid, sliced
- 1 teaspoon tomato paste
- 1 cup of coconut milk
- 1 teaspoon cayenne pepper
- ½ teaspoon salt

Method

1. Put all ingredients from the list above in the instant pot.

2. Close and seal the lid and cook the squid on manual (high pressure) for 20 minutes.

3. When the cooking time is finished, do the quick pressure release.

4. Serve the squid with coconut milk gravy.

   Nutritional info per serve: calories 326, fat 21.3, fiber 2, carbs 9.8, protein 25.5

Cod under the Bagel Spices Crust

Prep time: 10 minutes | **Cook time:** 10 minutes | **Yield:** 2 servings

Ingredients

- 6 oz cod fillet
- 1 tablespoon bagel spices
- 1 teaspoon olive oil
- 1 teaspoon butter

Method

1. Cut the cod fillet into 2 servings and sprinkle the bagel spices generously.

2. Then melt the butter in the instant pot. Add olive oil and stir gently.

3. Put the prepared cod fillets in the hot oil mixture and cook for 3.5 minutes per side on saute mode.

4. After this, close the lid and cook the fish on saute mode for 3 minutes.

   Nutritional info per serve: calories 133, fat 5, fiber 1.8, carbs 6.3, protein 16.7

Cioppino Stew

Prep time: 10 minutes | **Cook time:** 2 minutes | **Yield:** 4 servings

Ingredients

- 7 oz scallops
- 4 oz shrimps, peeled
- 1 tablespoon Italian seasonings
- ½ teaspoon minced garlic
- 1 cup beef broth
- 1 teaspoon tomato paste

Method

1. Put all ingredients in the instant pot and mix up gently with the help of the spoon.

2. Close and seal the lid. Cook the stew on manual mode (high pressure) for 2 minutes. Allow the natural pressure release for 5 minutes.

   Nutritional info per serve: calories 99, fat 2.3, fiber 0.1, carbs 2.6, protein 16.1

Ginger Cod

Prep time: 10 minutes | **Cook time:** 20 minutes | **Yield:** 2 servings

Ingredients

- 1 teaspoon ginger paste
- 8 oz cod fillet, chopped
- 1 tablespoon coconut oil
- ¼ cup of coconut milk

Method

1. Melt the coconut oil in the instant pot on saute mode.

2. Then add ginger paste and coconut milk and bring the mixture to boil.

3. Add chopped cod and saute the meal for 12 minutes. Stir the fish cubes with the help of the spatula from time to time.

   Nutritional info per serve: calories 222, fat 15, fiber 0.8, carbs 2.3, protein 21

Cinnamon Prawns

Prep time: 5 minutes | **Cook time:** 6 minutes | **Yield:** 2 servings

Ingredients

- 1 teaspoon ground cinnamon
- 12 oz prawns
- 1 teaspoon butter
- ½ cup cream

Method

1. Set the "Saute" mode and toss the butter in the instant pot bowl. Melt it.

2. Then add prawns and sprinkle them with the ground cinnamon. Stir well and cook for 3 minutes.

3. After this, add cream and lock the instant pot lid. Cook the meal for 3 minutes (QR).

   Nutritional info per serve: calories 260, fat 8.1, fiber 0.6, carbs 5.4, protein 39.3

Vegan

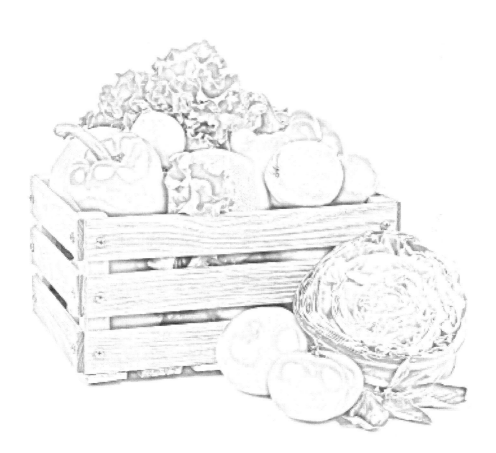

Spiced Cauliflower Head

Prep time: 15 minutes | **Cook time:** 17 minutes | **Yield:** 4 servings

Ingredients

- 13 oz cauliflower head
- 1 tablespoon avocado oil
- 1 tablespoon coconut cream
- 1 teaspoon ground turmeric
- 1 teaspoon ground paprika
- ½ teaspoon salt
- ½ teaspoon ground cumin
- 1 cup of water

Method

1. Pour water in the instant pot and insert the steamer rack.
2. In the mixing bowl, mix up avocado oil, coconut cream, ground turmeric, paprika, salt, and ground cumin.
3. Carefully brush the cauliflower head with a coconut cream mixture.
4. Sprinkle the remaining coconut cream mixture over the cauliflower.
5. Transfer the vegetable on the steamer rack.
6. Close and seal the lid.
7. Cook the cauliflower on manual mode (high pressure) for 7 minutes.
8. When the time is finished, allow the natural pressure release for 10 minutes.

Nutritional info per serve: calories 41, fat 1.6, fiber 2.9, carbs 6.1, protein 2.1

Teriyaki Eggplants

Prep time: 10 minutes | **Cook time:** 6 minutes | **Yield:** 6 servings

Ingredients

- 3 eggplants, trimmed
- 2 tablespoons keto teriyaki
- 2 tablespoons sesame oil
- ½ teaspoon ground ginger
- ½ teaspoon sesame seeds

Method

1. Heat up sesame oil in saute mode for 2 minutes.
2. Meanwhile, slice the eggplants and sprinkle them with teriyaki, ground ginger, and sesame seeds.
3. Arrange the eggplant slices in the instant pot bowl in one layer and cook them on saute mode for 2 minutes from each side.

Nutritional info per serve: calories 116, fat 5.2, fiber 9.7, carbs 17.2, protein 3.1

Tempeh Satay

Prep time: 5 minutes | **Cook time:** 4 minutes | **Yield:** 6 servings

Ingredients

- 15 oz tempeh
- 1 tablespoon coconut aminos
- ½ teaspoon harissa
- 1 tablespoon almond butter

Method

1. Chop the tempeh into cubes.
2. Then put the almond butter and harissa in the instant pot and melt it on saute mode.
3. Add chopped tempeh and coconut aminos.
4. Cook the meal on saute mode for 2 minutes – for 1 minute from each side.

Nutritional info per serve: calories 157, fat 9.2, fiber 0.3, carbs 7.8, protein 13.7

Vegan Pepperoni

Prep time: 20 minutes | **Cook time:** 4 minutes | **Yield:** 6 servings

Ingredients

- ½ cup nutritional yeast
- 1 teaspoon smoked paprika
- 1 teaspoon garlic powder
- ½ teaspoon salt
- ½ cup coconut flour
- 1 tablespoon almond butter, melted
- 4 tablespoons water
- 1 cup water, for cooking

Method

1. Blend together nutritional yeast, smoked paprika, garlic powder, salt, coconut flour, almond butter, and 4 tablespoons of water.
2. Then transfer the mixture in the sausage link or foil bag. Make the shape of pepperoni. Secure the ends of the pepperoni.
3. Pour water in the instant pot.
4. Then place the pepperoni in the water.
5. Close and seal the lid.
6. Cook the meal on manual (high pressure) for 4 minutes.
7. Allow the natural pressure release for 10 minutes.
8. Then cool the cooked pepperoni well and slice it.

Nutritional info per serve: calories 106, fat 3.3, fiber 7.8, carbs 13.8, protein 8.2

Parm Zucchini Noodles

Prep time: 10 minutes | **Cook time:** 5 minutes | **Yield:** 2 servings

Ingredients

- 1 large zucchini
- 1 garlic clove, diced
- 1 tablespoon butter
- 3 oz Parmesan, grated
- ½ teaspoon chili flakes

Method

1. Trim the zucchini and make the spirals from it with the help of the spiralizer.
2. Then toss the butter in the instant pot and melt it on saute mode.
3. Add garlic and chili flakes and cook the ingredients for 2 minutes.
4. After this, add zucchini spirals and cook them for 2 minutes.
5. Add grated Parmesan and mix up the meal well. Cook it for 1 minute more.

Nutritional info per serve: calories 216, fat 15.2, fiber 1.8, carbs 7.5, protein 15.8

Tofu Quiche

Prep time: 10 minutes | **Cook time:** 8 minutes | **Yield:** 4 servings

Ingredients

8 oz tofu

- ½ cup mushrooms, chopped, fried
- 1 teaspoon nutritional yeast
- 2 tablespoons almond flour
- 1 teaspoon coconut milk
- 1 teaspoon dried dill
- ¼ teaspoon salt
- 1 cup water, for cooking

Method

1. Chop tofu and mix it up with mushrooms, nutritional yeast, almond flour, coconut milk, dried dill, and salt.
2. Then place the mixture in the baking pan and flatten in the shape of the quiche.
3. Pour water in the instant pot and insert the steamer rack.
4. Place the quiche on the rack and close the lid.
5. Cook the meal on manual mode (high pressure) for 8 minutes. Then make a quick pressure release.

Nutritional info per serve: calories 69, fat 4.4, fiber 1.3, carbs 2.6, protein 6.1

Cauliflower Tikka Masala

Prep time: 10 minutes | **Cook time:** 3 minutes | **Yield:** 6 servings

Ingredients

- 1-pound cauliflower, chopped
- 1 teaspoon garam masala
- 1 tablespoon coconut oil
- 1 teaspoon ground
- turmeric
- 3 oz scallions, chopped
- 1 cup of coconut milk
- ¼ cup crushed tomatoes

Method

1. Put all ingredients in the instant pot and mix them well.
2. Then close and seal the lid.
3. Cook the tikka masala for 3 minutes on manual mode (high pressure).
4. Then allow the natural pressure release for 5 minutes.
5. Shake the cooked meal well before serving.

Nutritional info per serve: calories 140, fat 12, fiber 3.6, carbs 8.3, protein 3

Kale Stir Fry

Prep time: 10 minutes | **Cook time:** 3 minutes | **Yield:** 4 servings

Ingredients

- 8 oz asparagus, chopped
- 2 cups kale, chopped
- 2 bell pepper, chopped
- ½ teaspoon minced
- ginger
- 1 tablespoon avocado oil
- 1 teaspoon apple cider vinegar
- ½ cup of water

Method

1. In the instant pot baking pan, mix up together chopped kale, asparagus, bell pepper, minced ginger, apple cider vinegar, and avocado oil.
2. Then pour water in the instant pot.
3. Insert the steamer rack and place the mold with a kale mixture on it.
4. Close and seal the lid and cook the kale stir fry for 3 minutes on manual mode (high pressure). Make a quick pressure release.

Nutritional info per serve: calories 53, fat 0.7, fiber 2.7, carbs 10.6, protein 2.9

Thyme Cabbage

Prep time: 10 minutes | **Cook time:** 5 minutes | **Yield:** 4 servings

Ingredients

- 1-pound white cabbage
- 1 teaspoon dried thyme
- 2 tablespoons butter
- 1 cup of water
- ½ teaspoon salt

Method

1. Cut the white cabbage on medium size petals.
2. Then sprinkle it with dried thyme, butter, and salt.
3. Put the cabbage petals in the instant pot pan.
4. After this, pour water and insert the steamer rack in the instant pot.
5. Put the pan with cabbage on the rack and close the lid.
6. Cook the meal on manual mode (high pressure) for 5 minutes. Make a quick pressure release.

Nutritional info per serve: calories 80, fat 5.9, fiber 2.9, carbs 6.7, protein 1.5

Chives Mushrooms

Prep time: 10 minutes | **Cook time:** 3 minutes | **Yield:** 2 servings

Ingredients

1 cup cremini mushrooms, sliced

2 tablespoons chives, chopped

1 tablespoon sesame oil

1 teaspoon ranch seasonings

1 cup of water

Method

1. In the mixing bowl, mix up mushrooms, chives, sesame oil, and ranch seasonings.
2. Then pour water and insert the steamer rack in the instant pot.
3. Put the mushroom mixture in the baking pan and transfer it on the steamer rack.
4. Cook the meal on manual mode (high pressure) for 3 minutes.
5. When the time is finished, make a quick pressure release.

Nutritional info per serve: calories 70, fat 6.9, fiber 0.3, carbs 1.6, protein 1

Cauliflower Gnocchi

Prep time: 10 minutes | **Cook time:** 2 minutes | **Yield:** 4 servings

Ingredients

- 2 cups cauliflower, boiled
- 1 teaspoon salt
- ½ cup almond flour
- 1 tablespoon sesame oil
- 1 cup of water

Method

1. Mash the cauliflower until you get puree and mix it up with salt, almond flour, and sesame oil.
2. Then make the log from the cauliflower dough and cut it on small pieces.
3. Pour water in the instant pot.
4. Add gnocchi. Close and seal the lid.
5. Cook the meal on manual mode (high pressure) for 2 minutes.
6. Then allow the natural pressure release and open the lid.
7. Remove the cooked gnocchi from the water.

Nutritional info per serve: calories 127, fat 10.1, fiber 2.8, carbs 5.7, protein 4

Spiced Broccoli

Prep time: 10 minutes | **Cook time:** 4 minutes | **Yield:** 4 servings

Ingredients

- 2 cups broccoli florets
- 1 tablespoon lemon juice
- 1 teaspoon lemon zest, grated
- ½ teaspoon chili powder
- 1 tablespoon ground paprika
- 1 cup of water
- 1 teaspoon olive oil

Method

1. Pour water in the instant pot and insert the rack.
2. Put broccoli, lemon juice, lemon zest, chili powder, ground paprika, and olive oil in the baking pan and shake gently.
3. Then place the pan on the rack.
4. Close and seal the lid.
5. Cook the broccoli for 4 minutes on manual mode (high pressure).
6. Then make a quick pressure release.

Nutritional info per serve: calories 33, fat 1.6, fiber 2, carbs 4.3, protein 1.6

Beet Hummus

Prep time: 10 minutes | **Cook time:** 35 minutes | **Yield:** 4 servings

Ingredients

- 8 oz beets, peeled
- 1 teaspoon tahini paste
- ½ teaspoon harissa
- 1 tablespoon lemon juice
- 2 tablespoons olive oil
- ½ teaspoon salt
- 2 cups of water

Method

1. Put beets and water in the instant pot.
2. Cook the vegetables on manual mode (high pressure) for 35 minutes.
3. Then make a quick pressure release and open the lid.
4. Chop the beets and put them in the blender.
5. Add tahini paste, harissa, lemon juice, olive oil, and salt.
6. Blend the mixture until smooth.
7. Transfer the cooked hummus in the bowl.

Nutritional info per serve: calories 95, fat 7.9, fiber 1.3, carbs 6.2, protein 1.2

Jicama Mash

Prep time: 10 minutes | **Cook time:** 8 minutes | **Yield:** 4 servings

Ingredients

- 1-pound jicama, peeled, chopped
- 1 tablespoon almond butter
- 1 tablespoon chives, chopped
- ½ cup of coconut milk

Method

1. Put all ingredients from the list above in the instant pot.
2. Close and seal the lid.
3. Cook the jicama for 8 minutes on manual mode (high pressure), make quick pressure release.
4. Then transfer the mixture in the blender and blend until smooth.

Nutritional info per serve: calories 137, fat 9.5, fiber 6.6, carbs 12.4, protein 2.4

Zucchini Fritters

Prep time: 15 minutes | **Cook time:** 10 minutes | **Yield:** 4 servings

Ingredients

- 2 large zucchinis, grated
- 1 teaspoon ground flax meal
- 1 daikon, diced
- 1 egg, beaten
- 1 tablespoon coconut oil
- 1 teaspoon salt

Method

1. In the mixing bowl, mix up grated zucchini, ground flax meal, daikon, egg, and salt.
2. Make the fritters from the zucchini mixture.
3. After this, melt the coconut oil on saute mode.
4. Put the zucchini fritters in the hot oil and cook them for 4 minutes from each side or until they are golden brown.

Nutritional info per serve: calories 76, fat 4.9, fiber 2.1, carbs 6.3, protein 3.6

Sesame Zoodle Salad

Prep time: 10 minutes | **Cook time:** 3 minutes | **Yield:** 6 servings

Ingredients

- 2 large zucchinis, trimmed
- 1 teaspoon sesame seeds
- ¼ teaspoon chili flakes
- 1 tablespoon coconut aminos
- ¼ cup chicken broth
- 1 teaspoon sesame oil
- 1 tablespoon scallions, chopped

Method

1. Make the noodles from the zucchini using the spiralizer.
2. Then put them in the instant pot and add chicken broth.
3. Saute the zucchini zoodles for 3 minutes and transfer in the serving bowls.
4. Sprinkle the meal with sesame seeds, chili flakes, coconut aminos, sesame oil, and scallions.
5. Gently stir the zoodles.

Nutritional info per serve: calories 31, fat 1.3, fiber 1.3, carbs 4.3, protein 1.6

Mashed Turnips

Prep time: 10 minutes | **Cook time:** 5 minutes | **Yield:** 4 servings

Ingredients

- 2 cups turnips, peeled, chopped
- 3 cups of water
- 1 tablespoon coconut
- milk
- 1 teaspoon salt
- 1 oz tempeh, shredded

Method

1. Put turnips, water, and salt in the instant pot.
2. Close and seal the lid.
3. Cook the turnip on manual mode (high pressure) for 5 minutes. Make a quick pressure release.
4. Then open the lid and transfer the turnip in the blender.
5. Add tempeh and coconut milk.
6. Blend the meal until it is smooth.
7. Transfer the cooked turnips in the serving bowls.

Nutritional info per serve: calories 49, fat 1.7, fiber 1.6, carbs 6.9, protein 2.2

Keto Bread

Prep time: 15 minutes | **Cook time:** 30 minutes | **Yield:** 4 servings

Ingredients

- 4 eggs, beaten
- 1 teaspoon baking powder
- 1 cup almond flour
- 2 tablespoons chia
- seeds
- 1/3 cup coconut milk
- 1 teaspoon coconut oil, melted
- 1 cup of water

Method

1. Put all ingredients except water in the mixing bowl and knead the dough.
2. Then place the dough in the baking pan.
3. Pour water and insert the steamer rack in the instant pot.
4. Put the pan with dough on the steamer rack and close the lid.
5. Cook the bread on manual mode (high pressure) for 30 minutes.
6. Then make a quick pressure release.
7. Open the lid and let the cooked bread cool to room temperature.
8. Remove it from the pan and slice.

Nutritional info per serve: calories 322, fat 25.8, fiber 5.9, carbs 11, protein 13.2

Southern Okra

Prep time: 5 minutes | **Cook time:** 4 minutes | **Yield:** 2 servings

Ingredients

- ½ teaspoon Erythritol
- 1 teaspoon almond flour
- 1 cup okra, sliced
- 1 teaspoon coconut
- oil
- ½ tomato, chopped
- ½ bell pepper, chopped
- ½ cup of water

Method

1. Put all ingredients in the instant pot.
2. Close and seal the lid.
3. Then cook the meal on manual mode (high pressure) for 4 minutes.
4. When the time is finished, make a quick pressure release and transfer the meal on the plates.

Nutritional info per serve: calories 60, fat 3.2, fiber 2.3, carbs 6.9, protein 1.7

Summer Squash Gratin

Prep time: 15 minutes | **Cook time:** 10 minutes | **Yield:** 4 servings

Ingredients

- 2 zucchinis, sliced
- ½ cup of coconut milk
- 3 oz tofu, shredded
- 1 teaspoon chili flakes
- ½ teaspoon dried dill
- 1 teaspoon coconut oil
- 1 cup water, for cooking

Method

1. Grease the gratin mold with coconut oil.
2. Then place the sliced zucchini inside.
3. Add coconut milk, tofu, chili flakes, and dried dill.
4. Cover the gratin with foil and place it on the steamer rack.
5. Pour water in the instant pot.
6. Then transfer the steamer rack with gratin in the instant pot and close the lid.
7. Cook the gratin on manual mode (high pressure) for 10 minutes.
8. When the time is finished, allow the natural pressure release for 10 minutes.

Nutritional info per serve: calories 110, fat 9.4, fiber 2, carbs 5.4, protein 3.7

Scallions&Olives Salad

Prep time: 5 minutes | **Cook time:** 4 minutes | **Yield:** 2 servings

Ingredients

- 4 oz scallions, sliced
- 1 teaspoon coconut oil
- ½ teaspoon Splenda
- ½ cup olives, sliced
- 1 teaspoon sesame oil
- 1 tablespoon fresh parsley, chopped

Method

1. Put the sliced scallions and coconut oil in the instant pot.
2. Saute it for 4 minutes or until the scallions is light brown.
3. Then transfer it in the salad bowl.
4. Add sliced olives, parsley, and sesame oil. Stir the salad.

   Nutritional info per serve: calories 102, fat 8.3, fiber 2.6, carbs 7.4, protein 1.4

Falafel Salad

Prep time: 20 minutes | **Cook time:** 10 minutes | **Yield:** 4 servings

Ingredients

- 2 cups lettuce, chopped
- 1 cucumber, chopped
- 1 tablespoon olive oil
- 1 teaspoon lemon juice
- ½ teaspoon cayenne pepper
- 1 cup cauliflower, shredded
- 1 egg, beaten
- 1/3 cup coconut flour
- 1 teaspoon lemon zest, grated
- 2 tablespoons coconut oil

Method

1. Make the falafel: mix up grated lemon zest, coconut flour, egg, and cauliflower.
2. Then make the small balls (falafel).
3. Melt the coconut oil in the instant pot on saute mode and add falafel. Place them in one layer,
4. Cook the falafel balls on saute mode for 3-4 minutes per side or until they are golden brown.
5. Meanwhile, in the salad bowl, mix up lettuce, cucumber, olive oil, lemon juice, and cayenne pepper. Shake the salad well.
6. Then top it with the cooked falafel.

   Nutritional info per serve: calories 174, fat 13.3, fiber 5.3, carbs 11.2, protein 4.6

Broccoli Rice Bowl

Prep time: 10 minutes | **Cook time:** 1 minute | **Yield:** 2 servings

Ingredients

- 1 ½ cup broccoli, shredded
- ½ teaspoon salt
- ½ teaspoon ground turmeric
- 2 tablespoons cream cheese
- 1 cup water, for cooking

Method

1. Pour water and insert the steamer rack in the instant pot.
2. Put the broccoli shred in the bowl and transfer it in the steamer rack.
3. Close and seal the lid and cook it on manual mode (high pressure) for 1 minute + quick pressure release.
4. Transfer the cooked broccoli in the bowl and add salt, turmeric, and cream cheese.
5. Stir it well.

   Nutritional info per serve: calories 60, fat 3.8, fiber 1.9, carbs 5.2, protein 2.7

Low Carb Budha Bowl

Prep time: 10 minutes | **Cook time:** 5 minutes | **Yield:** 2 servings

Ingredients

- ½ cup cauliflower, chopped
- ½ cup mushrooms, chopped
- 4 oz bok choy, chopped
- 1 tablespoon avocado
- oil
- ½ teaspoon salt
- 1 tablespoon lemon juice
- 1 cup water, for cooking

Method

1. Pour water and insert the steamer in the instant pot.
2. Put all vegetables in the steamer; close and seal the lid.
3. Cook the ingredients on steam mode for 5 minutes. Then do the quick pressure release.
4. After this, transfer the cooked vegetables in the serving bowls and sprinkle with salt, lemon juice, and avocado oil.

   Nutritional info per serve: calories 29, fat 1.1, fiber 1.7, carbs 3.7, protein 2.1

Zucchini Hasselback

Prep time: 15 minutes | **Cook time:** 8 minutes | **Yield:** 2 servings

Ingredients

- 2 zucchinis, trimmed
- 2 teaspoons olive oil
- ½ teaspoon white pepper
- ½ teaspoon salt
- 1 cup water, for cooking

Method

1. Cut the zucchinis in the shape of the Hasselback and sprinkle with white pepper, salt, and olive oil.
2. Then place the vegetables on the rack and place it in the instant pot. Add water.
3. Close and seal the lid and cook the meal on manual mode (high pressure) for 8 minutes.
4. Make a quick pressure release and remove the zucchinis from the instant pot.

Nutritional info per serve: calories 73, fat 5, fiber 2.3, carbs 6.9, protein 2.4

Portobello Cheese Sandwiches

Prep time: 15 minutes | **Cook time:** 6 minutes | **Yield:** 2 servings

Ingredients

- 4 Portobello mushrooms caps
- ¼ teaspoon minced garlic
- 1 tablespoon olive oil
- 2 Cheddar cheese slices
- 1 cup water, for cooking

Method

1. In the shallow bowl mix up garlic and olive oil.
2. Brush the mushrooms with garlic mixture and place them on the trivet.
3. Pour water in the instant pot. Transfer the trivet with mushroom caps inside.
4. Close and seal the lid and cook the vegetables for 6 minutes on manual mode (high pressure).
5. Then make a quick pressure release and open the lid.
6. Place the cheese slices on 2 mushroom caps and cover them with remaining mushroom to get the shape of sandwiches.

Nutritional info per serve: calories 188, fat 16.3, fiber 0, carbs 1.9, protein 8.4

Turnip Roast

Prep time: 10 minutes | **Cook time:** 10 minutes | **Yield:** 2 servings

Ingredients

- 2 turnips, peeled, chopped
- ½ teaspoon ground paprika
- 1 tablespoon olive oil
- ¼ teaspoon salt
- ¼ teaspoon ground black pepper

Method

1. Sprinkle the chopped turnip with ground paprika, salt, and ground black pepper.
2. Then heat up olive oil in the instant pot on saute mode and add chopped turnip.
3. Cook the turnip on saute mode for 3 minutes from each side.
4. Then close the lid and saute it for 4 minutes more.

Nutritional info per serve: calories 97, fat 7.1, fiber 2.3, carbs 8.5, protein 1.1

Butter Chanterelle Mushrooms

Prep time: 10 minutes | **Cook time:** 15 minutes | **Yield:** 4 servings

Ingredients

- 14 oz chanterelle mushrooms, chopped
- ½ cup heavy cream
- 3 tablespoons butter
- 1 teaspoon salt
- ½ teaspoon dried thyme

Method

1. Melt the butter in the instant pot on saute mode and add chanterelle mushrooms.
2. Add dried thyme and salt and saute the vegetables for 5 minutes.
3. Then stir them well and add heavy cream. Close and seal the lid.
4. Cook the mushrooms on manual mode (high pressure) for 10 minutes.
5. Then do the quick pressure release.

Nutritional info per serve: calories 130, fat 14.2, fiber 0.1, carbs 0.7, protein 0.6

Portobello Steak

Prep time: 7 minutes | **Cook time:** 10 minutes |
Yield: 2 servings

Ingredients

- 7 oz Portobello mushroom cap
- 1 teaspoon butter
- ¼ teaspoon meat seasonings
- ¼ cup ricotta cheese

Method

1. Rub the mushrooms with meat seasonings and put in the instant pot.

2. Add butter and cook the vegetables on saute mode for 3 minutes from each side.

3. Then add ricotta cheese and cook mushroom steaks for 4 minutes more.

   Nutritional info per serve: calories 85, fat 4.6, fiber 1.5, carbs 6.6, protein 6

Herbed Radish

Prep time: 5 minutes | **Cook time:** 10 minutes |
Yield: 2 servings

Ingredients

- 2 cups radish, roughly chopped
- 2 tablespoons butter
- 1 teaspoon Italian seasonings
- ¼ teaspoon dried rosemary
- ¼ cup of water

Method

1. Put all ingredients in the instant pot and mix them up.

2. Saute the meal for 10 minutes, Stir it with the help of the spatula every 3 minutes.

Nutritional info per serve: calories 128, fat 12.4, fiber 1.9, carbs 4.3, protein 0.9

Desserts

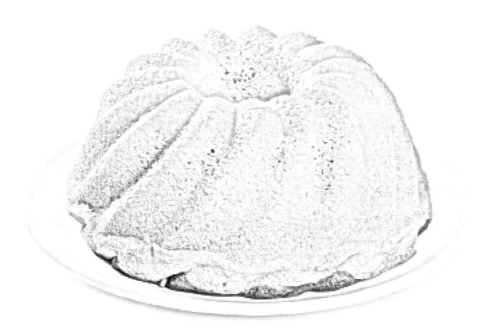

Pumpkin Pie Spices Cheesecake

Prep time: 10 minutes | **Cook time:** 40 minutes | **Yield:** 8 servings

Ingredients

- 3 tablespoons almond flour
- 1 tablespoon butter, softened
- 3 tablespoons Erythritol
- 1 cup cream cheese
- 1 egg, beaten
- ¼ cup of coconut milk
- 1 teaspoon pumpkin pie spices
- 1 cup water, for cooking

Method

1. In the mixing bowl mix up almond flour, butter, and 1 tablespoon of Erythritol. Knead the dough.
2. Transfer the dough in the cheesecake mold and flatten it to get the pie crust shape. Place it in the freezer for 10 minutes.
3. Meanwhile, put the cream cheese, egg, coconut milk, pumpkin pie spices, and remaining Erythritol in the mixing bowl. Mix the mixture until smooth with the help of the hand mixer.
4. Pour the cream cheese mixture over the frozen pie crust, flatten it well.
5. Pour water and insert the steamer rack in the instant pot and put the cheesecake on it.
6. Close and seal the lid.
7. Cook it on manual (high pressure) for 30 minutes. Make a quick pressure release.

Nutritional info per serve: calories 156, fat 15.2, fiber 0.5, carbs 7.6, protein 3.6

Anise Hot Chocolate

Prep time: 10 minutes | **Cook time:** 2 minutes | **Yield:** 3 servings

Ingredients

- 1 tablespoon cocoa powder
- 1 tablespoon Erythritol
- ¼ cup heavy cream
- ½ cup of coconut milk
- ½ teaspoon ground anise

Method

1. Put all ingredients in the instant pot bowl. Stir them well until you get a smooth liquid.
2. Close and seal the lid.
3. Cook the hot chocolate on manual (high pressure) for 2 minutes. Then allow the natural pressure release for 5 minutes.

Nutritional info per serve: calories 131, fat 13.5, fiber 1.4, carbs 8.5, protein 1.5

Daikon Cake

Prep time: 10 minutes | **Cook time:** 45 minutes | **Yield:** 12 servings

Ingredients

- 5 eggs, beaten
- ½ cup heavy cream
- 1 cup almond flour
- 1 daikon, diced
- 1 teaspoon ground cinnamon
- 2 tablespoon Erythritol
- 1 tablespoon butter, melted
- 1 cup water, for cooking

Method

1. In the mixing bowl, mix up eggs, heavy cream, almond flour, ground cinnamon, and Erythritol.
2. When the mixture is smooth, add daikon and stir it carefully with the help of the spatula.
3. Pour the mixture in the cake pan.
4. Then pour water and insert the steamer rack in the instant pot.
5. Place the cake in the instant pot.
6. Close and seal the lid.
7. Cook the cake in manual mode (high pressure) for 45 minutes. Make a quick pressure release.

Nutritional info per serve: calories 67, fat 5.8, fiber 0.4, carbs 3.6, protein 3

Almond Pie

Prep time: 15 minutes | **Cook time:** 41 minutes | **Yield:** 8 servings

Ingredients

- 1 cup almond flour
- ½ cup of coconut milk
- 1 teaspoon vanilla extract
- 2 tablespoons butter,
- softened
- 1 tablespoon Truvia
- ¼ cup coconut, shredded
- 1 cup water, for cooking

Method

1. In the mixing bowl, mix up almond flour, coconut milk, vanilla extract, butter, Truvia, and shredded coconut.
2. When the mixture is smooth, transfer it in the baking pan and flatten.
3. Pour water and insert the steamer rack in the instant pot.
4. Put the baking pan with cake on the rack. Close and seal the lid.
5. Cook the dessert on manual mode (high pressure) for 41 minutes. Allow the natural pressure release for 10 minutes.

Nutritional info per serve: calories 90, fat 9.1, fiber 0.9, carbs 2.6, protein 1.2

Coconut Cupcakes

Prep time: 15 minutes | **Cook time:** 10 minutes | **Yield:** 6 servings

Ingredients

- 4 eggs, beaten
- 4 tablespoons coconut milk
- 4 tablespoons coconut flour
- ½ teaspoon vanilla extract
- 2 tablespoons Erythritol
- 1 teaspoon baking powder
- 1 cup water, for cooking

Method

1. In the mixing bowl, mix up eggs, coconut milk, coconut flour, vanilla extract, Erythritol, and baking powder.
2. Then pour the batter in the cupcake molds.
3. Pour water and insert the steamer rack in the instant pot.
4. Place the cupcakes on the rack. Close and seal the lid.
5. Cook the cupcakes for 10 minutes on manual mode (high pressure).
6. Then allow the natural pressure release for 5 minutes.

Nutritional info per serve: calories 86, fat 5.8, fiber 2.2, carbs 9.2, protein 4.6

Chocolate Mousse

Prep time: 10 minutes | **Cook time:** 4 minutes | **Yield:** 1 serving

Ingredients

- 1 egg yolk
- 1 teaspoon Erythritol
- 1 teaspoon of cocoa powder
- 2 tablespoons coconut milk
- 1 tablespoon cream cheese
- 1 cup water, for cooking

Method

1. Pour water and insert the steamer rack in the instant pot.
2. Then whisk the egg yolk with Erythritol.
3. When the mixture turns into lemon color, add coconut milk, cream cheese, and cocoa powder. Whisk the mixture until smooth.
4. Then pour it in the glass jar and place it on the steamer rack.
5. Close and seal the lid.
6. Cook the dessert on manual (high pressure) for 4 minutes. Make a quick pressure release.

Nutritional info per serve: calories 162, fat 15.4, fiber 1.2, carbs 3.5, protein 4.5

Lime Muffins

Prep time: 10 minutes | **Cook time:** 15 minutes | **Yield:** 6 servings

Ingredients

- 1 teaspoon lime zest
- 1 tablespoon lemon juice
- 1 teaspoon baking powder
- 1 cup almond flour
- 2 eggs, beaten
- 1 tablespoon swerve
- ¼ cup heavy cream
- 1 cup water, for cooking

Method

1. In the mixing bowl, mix up lemon juice, baking powder, almond flour, eggs, swerve, and heavy cream.
2. When the muffin batter is smooth, add lime zest and mix it up.
3. Fill the muffin molds with batter.
4. Then pour water and insert the rack in the instant pot.
5. Place the muffins on the rack. Close and seal the lid.
6. Cook the muffins on manual (high pressure) for 15 minutes.
7. Then allow the natural pressure release.

Nutritional info per serve: calories 153, fat 12.2, fiber 2.1, carbs 5.1, protein 6

Pecan Pralines

Prep time: 15 minutes | **Cook time:** 7 minutes | **Yield:** 4 servings

Ingredients

- 4 pecans
- 4 teaspoons coconut oil
- 1 teaspoon of cocoa powder
- 1 teaspoon Erythritol

Method

1. Heat up the instant pot on saute mode.
2. Then add coconut oil and cocoa powder. Saute the mixture until it is smooth and homogenous.
3. Meanwhile, line the tray with baking paper.
4. Put the pecans on the baking paper.
5. Pour the hot coconut oil mixture over the pecans. Refrigerate the pralines for 10-15 minutes.

Nutritional info per serve: calories 138, fat 14.6, fiber 1.6, carbs 3.5, protein 1.6

Vanilla Hot Drink

Prep time: 2 minutes | **Cook time:** 7 minutes | **Yield:** 2 servings

Ingredients

- 1 cup almond milk
- 1 teaspoon butter
- 1 teaspoon vanilla extract
- 1 teaspoon erythritol
- 1 tablespoon cocoa powder

Method

1. Transfer all the ingredients into the instant pot bowl.
2. Set the "Saute" and start to cook the hot chocolate.
3. Saute the hot chocolate until it starts to boil. (around 10 minutes).

   Nutritional info per serve: calories 29, fat 3.8, fiber 0.8, carbs 4.3, protein 1

Blueberry Muffins

Prep time: 15 minutes | **Cook time:** 14 minutes | **Yield:** 3 servings

Ingredients

- ¼ cup blueberries
- ¼ teaspoon baking powder
- 1 teaspoon apple cider vinegar
- 4 teaspoons butter, melted
- 2 eggs, beaten
- 1 cup coconut flour
- 2 tablespoons Erythritol
- 1 cup water, for cooking

Method

1. In the mixing bowl, mix up baking powder, apple cider vinegar, butter, eggs, coconut flour, and Erythritol.
2. When the batter is smooth, add blueberries. Stir well.
3. Put the muffin batter in the muffin molds.
4. After this, pour water and insert the steamer rack in the instant pot.
5. Then place the muffins on the rack. Close and seal the lid.
6. Cook the muffins on manual mode (high pressure) for 14 minutes.
7. When the time is finished, allow the natural pressure release for 6 minutes.

   Nutritional info per serve: calories 95, fat 4.5, fiber 6.1, carbs 14.6, protein 3.4

Low Carb Brownie

Prep time: 15 minutes | **Cook time:** 15 minutes | **Yield:** 8 servings

Ingredients

- 1 cup coconut flour
- 1 tablespoon cocoa powder
- 1 tablespoon coconut oil
- 1 teaspoon vanilla extract
- 1 teaspoon baking powder
- 1 teaspoon apple cider vinegar
- 1/3 cup butter, melted
- 1 tablespoon Erythritol
- 1 cup water, for cooking

Method

1. In the mixing bowl, mix up Erythritol, melted butter, apple cider vinegar, baking powder, vanilla extract, coconut oil, cocoa powder, and coconut flour.
2. Whisk the mixture until smooth and pour it in the baking pan. Flatten the surface of the batter.
3. Pour water and insert the steamer rack in the instant pot.
4. Put the pan with brownie batter on the rack. Close and seal the lid.
5. Cook the brownie on manual mode (high pressure) for 15 minutes.
6. Then allow the natural pressure release for 5 minutes.
7. Cut the cooked brownies into the bars.

   Nutritional info per serve: calories 146, fat 11, fiber 6.2, carbs 12.6, protein 2.2

Vanilla Curd

Prep time: 5 minutes | **Cook time:** 5 minutes | **Yield:** 3 servings

Ingredients

- 4 egg yolks, whisked
- 2 tablespoon butter
- 1 tablespoon Erythritol
- ½ cup organic almond milk
- 1 teaspoon vanilla extract

Method

1. Set the instant pot in "Saute" mode and when the "Hot" is displayed – add butter.
2. Melt the butter but not boil it and add whisked egg yolks, almond milk, and vanilla extract.
3. Add Erythritol. Whisk the mixture.
4. Cook the meal on "Low" for 6 hours.

   Nutritional info per serve: calories 154, fat 14.1, fiber 0, carbs 7.3, protein 3.9

Crème Brule

Prep time: 25 minutes | **Cook time:** 10 minutes | **Yield:** 2 servings

Ingredients

- 1 cup heavy cream
- 5 egg yolks
- 2 tablespoons swerve
- 1 cup water, for cooking

Method

1. Whisk the egg yolks and swerve together.

2. Then add heavy cream and stir the mixture carefully.

3. Pour the mixture in ramekins and place them on the steamer rack.

4. Pour water in the instant pot. Add steamer rack with ramekins.

5. Close and seal the lid.

6. Cook crème Brule for 10 minutes – High pressure. Allow the natural pressure release for 15 minutes.

Nutritional info per serve: calories 347, fat 33.5, fiber 0, carbs 5.2, protein 8

Lava Cake

Prep time: 15 minutes | **Cook time:** 18 minutes | **Yield:** 4 servings

Ingredients

- 1 teaspoon baking powder
- 1 tablespoon cocoa powder
- 1 cup coconut cream
- 1/3 cup coconut flour
- 1 tablespoon almond flour
- 2 teaspoons Erythritol
- 1 tablespoon butter, melted
- 1 cup water, for cooking

Method

1. Whisk together baking powder, cocoa powder, coconut cream, coconut flour, almond flour, Erythritol, and butter.

2. Then pour the chocolate mixture in the baking cups.

3. Pour water in the instant pot. Insert the steamer rack.

4. Place the cups with cake mixture on the rack. Close and seal the lid.

5. Cook the lava cakes on manual (high pressure) for 4 minutes. Allow the natural pressure release for 5 minutes.

Nutritional info per serve: calories 218, fat 19.2, fiber 5.9, carbs 14.2, protein 3.4

Vanilla Pie

Prep time: 20 minutes | **Cook time:** 35 minutes | **Yield:** 12 servings

Ingredients

- 1 cup heavy cream
- 3 eggs, beaten
- 1 teaspoon vanilla extract
- ¼ cup Erythritol
- 1 cup coconut flour
- 1 tablespoon butter, melted
- 1 cup water, for cooking

Method

1. In the mixing bowl, mix up coconut flour, Erythritol, vanilla extract, eggs, and heavy cream.

2. Grease the baking pan with melted butter.

3. Pour the coconut mixture in the baking pan.

4. Pour water and insert the steamer rack in the instant pot.

5. Place the pie on the rack. Close and seal the lid.

6. Cook the pie on manual mode (high pressure) for 35 minutes.

7. Allow the natural pressure release for 10 minutes.

Nutritional info per serve: calories 100, fat 6.8, fiber 4, carbs 12.1, protein 2.9

Custard

Prep time: 10 minutes | **Cook time:** 7 minutes | **Yield:** 4 servings

Ingredients

- 6 eggs, beaten
- 1 cup heavy cream
- 1 teaspoon vanilla extract
- ¼ teaspoon ground nutmeg
- 2 tablespoons Erythritol
- 1 tablespoon coconut flour
- 1 cup water, for cooking

Method

1. Whisk the eggs and Erythritol until smooth.

2. Then add heavy cream, vanilla extract, ground nutmeg, and coconut flour.

3. Whisk the mixture well again.

4. Then pour it in the custard ramekins and cover with foil.

5. Pour water and insert the steamer rack in the instant pot.

6. Place the ramekins with custard on the rack. Close and seal the lid.

7. Cook the meal on manual (high pressure) for 7 minutes. Make a quick pressure release.

Nutritional info per serve: calories 209, fat 17.9, fiber 0.8, carbs 10.3, protein 9.2

Pecan Pie

Prep time: 20 minutes | **Cook time:** 25 minutes | **Yield:** 4 servings

Ingredients

- 2 tablespoons coconut oil
- 4 tablespoons almond flour
- 4 pecans, chopped
- 1 tablespoon
- Erythritol
- 2 tablespoons butter
- 1 tablespoon coconut flour
- 1 cup water, for cooking

Method

1. Make the pie crust: mix up coconut oil and almond flour in the bowl.
2. Then knead the dough and put it in the baking pan. Flatten the dough in the shape of the pie crust.
3. Then melt Erythritol, butter, and coconut flour.
4. When the mixture is liquid, add chopped pecans.
5. Pour water in the instant pot and insert the steamer rack.
6. Pour the butter-pecan mixture over the pie crust, flatten it and transfer on the steamer rack.
7. Cook the pecan pie on manual mode (high pressure) for 25 minutes.
8. Allow the natural pressure release for 10 minutes and cool the cooked pie well.

Nutritional info per serve: calories 257, fat 26.1, fiber 3, carbs 8.5, protein 3.3

Sweet Zucchini Crisps

Prep time: 6 minutes | **Cook time:** 8 minutes | **Yield:** 2 servings

Ingredients

- 1 tablespoon Erythritol
- 1 zucchini
- 1 tablespoon butter

Method

1. Slice the zucchini into thin rounds.
2. The heat up butter on saute mode. When the butter is hot, add zucchini slices and cook them for 4 minutes from each side or until they become light crispy.
3. Then sprinkle the cooked crisps with Erythritol and put on the paper towel for 10 minutes to cool.

Nutritional info per serve: calories 67, fat 5.9, fiber 1.1, carbs 3.3, protein 1.3

Vanilla Flan

Prep time: 10 minutes | **Cook time:** 8 minutes | **Yield:** 4 servings

Ingredients

- 4 egg whites
- 4 egg yolks
- ½ cup Erythritol
- 7 oz heavy cream, whipped
- 3 tablespoons water
- 1 tablespoon butter
- ½ teaspoon vanilla extract
- 1 cup water, for cooking

Method

1. In the saucepan, heat up Erythritol and butter. When the mixture is smooth, leave it in a warm place.
2. Meanwhile, mix up water, heavy cream, egg whites, and egg yolks. Whisk the mixture.
3. Pour the Erythritol mixture in the flan ramekins and then add heavy cream mixture over the sweet mixture.
4. Pour water and insert the steamer rack in the instant pot.
5. Place the ramekins with flan on the rack. Close and seal the lid.
6. Cook the dessert on manual (high pressure) for 10 minutes. Then allow the natural pressure release for 10 minutes.
7. Cool the cooked flan for 25 minutes.

Nutritional info per serve: calories 269, fat 25.8, fiber 0, carbs 2.3, protein 7.4

Keto Soufflé

Prep time: 10 minutes | **Cook time:** 6 hours | **Yield:** 4 servings

Ingredients

- ½ cup of coconut milk
- 4 egg yolks
- 2 tablespoons Splenda
- 1 tablespoon almond flour
- 1 cup of water (for instant pot)

Method

1. Put coconut milk, egg yolk, Splenda, and almond flour in the blender.
2. Blend the mixture until smooth and pour it in the small ramekins.
3. Then pour water in the instant pot and place the ramekins with soufflé inside.
4. Close the lid and cook the dessert on "Low" for 6 hours.

Nutritional info per serve: calories 163, fat 12.5, fiber 0.9, carbs 8.7, protein 3.8

Mint Brownies

Prep time: 20 minutes | **Cook time:** 10 minutes | **Yield:** 4 servings

Ingredients

- 1 tablespoon cocoa powder
- 1 tablespoon Erythritol
- 2 egg yolks, whisked
- ¼ cup of coconut milk
- 1 teaspoon butter
- 1 teaspoon dried mint
- 3 tablespoons almond flour, gluten-free
- 1 cup of water (for instant pot)

Method

1. Pour coconut milk in the instant pot bowl and start to cook it on "saute" mode.
2. Add cocoa powder.
3. After this, add coconut milk and butter.
4. When the mixture is smooth – start to add whisked egg yolks gradually. Add almond flour.
5. Whisk the mixture without stopping.
6. Add Erythritol and mint. Whisk it all the time. Then flatten it.
7. Cook the dessert on "manual" mode for 10 minutes (QPR for 5 minutes).
8. Cut the dessert into bars.

Nutritional info per serve: calories 196, fat 17.8, fiber 3, carbs 10.3, protein 6.6

Pancake Bites

Prep time: 10 minutes | **Cook time:** 10 minutes | **Yield:** 4 servings

Ingredients

- 1 teaspoon apple cider vinegar
- 1 teaspoon vanilla extract
- 1 cup of coconut milk
- 1/3 cup coconut flour
- 1 tablespoon Erythritol
- ½ teaspoon baking powder
- 1 tablespoon coconut oil

Method

1. Melt the almond butter on saute mode.
2. Then mix up all the remaining ingredients in the mixing bowl.
3. Pour the small amount of pancake batter in the instant pot to get the small rounds.
4. Cook the pancake bites on saute mode for 1.5 minutes from each side.

Nutritional info per serve: calories 211, fat 18.7, fiber 5.3, carbs 14.2, protein 2.7

Fluffy Brulee

Prep time: 10 minutes | **Cook time:** 9 minutes | **Yield:** 3 servings

Ingredients

- 1 cup coconut cream
- 4 egg yolks
- 2 teaspoons
- Erythritol
- 1 cup of water (for instant pot)

Method

1. Whisk the egg yolk until you get the yellow color. Then add coconut cream and keep whisking the egg yolk mixture until smooth.
2. Add 1 teaspoon of Erythritol. Stir it well and transfer into the ramekins.
3. Pour 1 cup of water in the instant pot bowl. Place the steamer rack inside the instant pot.
4. Transfer the ramekins on the rack and wrap the top of ramekins with the foil.
5. Set the "Manual" mode (High pressure) and cook the dessert for 9 minutes.
6. Allow the natural pressure release for 15 minutes. Chill the dessert for 2 hours.

Nutritional info per serve: calories 256, fat 25.1, fiber 1.8, carbs 8.6, protein 5.4

Mug Muffins

Prep time: 10 minutes | **Cook time:** 8 minutes | **Yield:** 3 servings

Ingredients

- 1 teaspoon avocado oil
- 2 tablespoons coconut flour
- 1 tablespoon Erythritol
- ½ teaspoon vanilla
- extract
- ¼ teaspoon baking powder
- 1 tablespoon almond butter
- 1 cup of water (for instant pot)

Method

1. Brush the mugs with avocado oil
2. Mix up together all remaining the liquid ingredients and almond butter.
3. Add all the dry ingredients and stir the mixture with the help of the spoon.
4. When you get a smooth batter – transfer it into the prepared mugs.
5. Pour 1 cup of water in the instant pot and insert the steamer rack. Put the mugs on the rack and close the lid.
6. Cook the meal on "Manual" (High pressure) for 8 minutes. QPR for 5 minutes.

Nutritional info per serve: calories 58, fat 3.7, fiber 2.6, carbs 9.4, protein 2.3

Cocoa Cookie

Prep time: 15 minutes | **Cook time:** 25 minutes | **Yield:** 4 servings

Ingredients

- ½ cup coconut flour
- 3 tablespoons cream cheese
- 1 teaspoon of cocoa powder
- 1 tablespoon Erythritol
- ¼ teaspoon baking powder
- 1 teaspoon apple cider vinegar
- 1 tablespoon butter
- 1 cup water, for cooking

Method

1. Make the dough: mix up coconut flour, cream cheese, cocoa powder, Erythritol, baking powder, apple cider vinegar, and butter. Knead the dough,
2. Then transfer the dough in the baking pan and flatten it in the shape of a cookie.
3. Pour water and insert the steamer rack in the instant pot. Put the pan with a cookie in the instant pot. Close and seal the lid.
4. Cook the cookie on manual (high pressure) for 25 minutes. Make a quick pressure release. Cool the cookie well.

Nutritional info per serve: calories 113, fat 7.1, fiber 6.1, carbs 14.4, protein 2.7

Red Velvet Muffins

Prep time: 10 minutes | **Cook time:** 15 minutes | **Yield:** 2 servings

Ingredients

- ¼ teaspoon red food coloring
- 2 teaspoons butter
- ¼ teaspoon baking powder
- 1 teaspoon apple cider vinegar
- 4 tablespoons coconut flour
- 1 teaspoon vanilla extract
- 3 tablespoons heavy cream
- 1 cup water, for cooking

Method

1. In the mixing bowl, mix up red food coloring, butter, baking powder, apple cider vinegar, coconut flour, vanilla extract, and heavy cream.
2. Stir the mixture until it is smooth.
3. After this, pour the mixture in the muffin molds.
4. Pour water and insert the steamer rack in the instant pot. Place the muffin molds on the rack. Close and seal the lid.
5. Cook the muffins on manual (high pressure) for 15 minutes. Make a quick pressure release.

Nutritional info per serve: calories 179, fat 13.6, fiber 6, carbs 11.2, protein 2.5

Pecan Bites

Prep time: 20 minutes | **Cook time:** 8 minutes | **Yield:** 4 servings

Ingredients

- 2 pecans, crushed
- 1 tablespoon coconut oil, softened
- 1 egg, whisked
- ½ cup almond flour
- 1 tablespoon Erythritol
- ½ teaspoon vanilla extract
- ¼ cup of coconut milk
- ¾ teaspoon ground cinnamon
- ½ teaspoon sesame oil

Method

1. Spread the non-sticky springform mold with the sesame oil.
2. Then combine together the softened coconut oil, whisked egg, almond flour, vanilla extract, coconut milk, Erythritol, and ground cinnamon. Add pecans.
3. Check if all the ingredients are added and mix up the mixture until smooth.
4. Transfer the mixture in the prepared springform pan and flatten it well.
5. Place the pan in the instant pot and cover with the foil. Close the lid and cook the dessert on the "Manual" mode for 8 minutes (follow the directions of your instant pot). NPR for 15 minutes.
6. Cut the meal into bites.

Nutritional info per serve: calories 220, fat 20.3, fiber 2.8, carbs 9, .1protein 5.5

Sugar-Free Coconut Squares

Prep time: 15 minutes | **Cook time:** 4 minutes | **Yield:** 2 servings

Ingredients

- 1/3 cup coconut flakes
- 1 tablespoon butter
- 1 egg, beaten
- 1 cup water, for cooking

Method

1. Mix up together coconut flakes, butter, and egg.
2. Then put the mixture into the square shape mold and flatten well.
3. Pour water and insert the steamer rack in the instant pot. Put the mold with dessert on the rack. Close and seal the lid.
4. Cook the meal on manual mode (high pressure) for 4 minutes. Make a quick pressure release.
5. Cool the cooked dessert little and cut into the squares.

Nutritional info per serve: calories 130, fat 12.4, fiber 1.2, carbs 2.2, protein 3.3

Custard Tarts

Prep time: 10 minutes | **Cook time:** 20 minutes | **Yield:** 2 servings

Ingredients

- ¼ cup almond flour
- 1 tablespoon coconut oil
- 2 egg yolks
- ¼ cup of coconut milk
- 1 tablespoon Erythritol
- 1 teaspoon vanilla extract
- 1 cup water, for cooking

Method

1. Make the dough: mix up almond flour and coconut oil.

2. Then place the dough into 2 mini tart molds and flatten well in the shape of cups.

3. Pour water in the instant pot. Insert the steamer rack. Place the tart mold in the instant pot. Close and seal the lid.

4. Cook them for 3 minutes on Manual mode (high pressure). Make a quick pressure release.

5. Then whisk together vanilla extract, Erythritol, coconut milk, and egg yolks.

6. Pour the liquid in the tart molds and close the lid. Cook the dessert for 7 minutes on manual mode (high pressure).

7. Then allow the natural pressure release for 10 minutes more.

Nutritional info per serve: calories 208, fat 20.2, fiber 1, carbs 3.3, protein 4.1

Peanut Cheesecake

Prep time: 10 minutes | **Cook time:** 8 hours | **Yield:** 4 servings

Ingredients

- 1 cup cream cheese
- 4 eggs, beaten
- 1 teaspoon vanilla extract
- ¼ cup of coconut milk
- 1 teaspoon coconut
- oil
- 1 tablespoon erythritol
- 2 oz peanuts, chopped
- 1 cup water, for cooking

Method

1. Mix up together cream cheese, eggs, vanilla extract, coconut milk, coconut oil, Erythritol, and peanuts.

2. Then pour the liquid in the instant pot baking pan. Flatten the surface of the cheesecake if desired.

3. Then pour water in the instant pot and insert the mold with cheesecake. Close the lid and cook the dessert on "low" mode for 8 hours.

Nutritional info per serve: calories 393, fat 6.3, fiber 1.5, carbs 8.9, protein 13.9

Ramekin Red Cakes

Prep time: 10 minutes | **Cook time:** 15 minutes | **Yield:** 2 servings

Ingredients

- ¼ teaspoon red food coloring
- 2 teaspoons almond butter
- ¼ teaspoon baking powder
- 1 teaspoon lemon
- juice
- 4 tablespoons almond flour
- 3 tablespoons coconut cream
- 1 cup water, for cooking

Method

1. Mix up red food coloring, almond butter, baking powder, lemon juice, and almond flour.

2. Add coconut cream. Stir the mixture until it is smooth. After this, pour the mixture in the non-sticky ramekins.

3. Pour water and insert the steamer rack in the instant pot. Place the ramekins on the rack. Cook the muffins on manual (high pressure) for 15 minutes + quick pressure release.

Nutritional info per serve: calories 235, fat 21, fiber 3.6, carbs 7.6, protein 6.9

Avocado Bread

Prep time: 5 minutes | **Cook time:** 3 minutes | **Yield:** 4 servings

Ingredients

- 1 avocado, mashed
- ½ teaspoon baking powder
- ¼ teaspoon apple cider vinegar
- 1 teaspoon vanilla extract
- 1 tablespoon Erythritol
- 1 egg, whisked
- ¼ cup coconut cream
- ½ cup coconut flour
- 1 cup water (for instant pot)

Method

1. Combine together the baking powder, apple cider vinegar, vanilla extract, Erythritol, and whisked egg.

2. Add coconut cream and coconut flour. Add mashed avocado. Mix up the mixture until you get the homogenous texture.

3. Transfer the dough into the non-stick cake mold and flatten gently with the help of the spatula.

4. Wrap the mold in the aluminum foil.

5. Pour water in the instant pot and insert the steamer rack. Place the mold on the rack and close the lid. Cook the bread on the "Steam" mode for 20 minutes. Use the quick pressure release.

6. Chill the bread and remove it from the cake mold.

Nutritional info per serve: calories 216, fat 16, fiber 9.7, carbs 19.4, protein 4.7

Cinnamon Roll

Prep time: 15 minutes | **Cook time:** 20 minutes | **Yield:** 4 servings

Ingredients

- 1 tablespoon ground cinnamon
- 1 tablespoon butter, softened
- 2 tablespoons coconut oil
- 1 tablespoon Erythritol
- ½ cup almond flour
- ½ teaspoon baking powder
- 1 cup water, for cooking

Method

1. In the mixing bowl, mix up coconut oil, almond flour, and baking powder. Knead the dough. Then roll it up and grease with butter.

2. Then sprinkle the dough with Erythritol and ground cinnamon. Roll the dough into a log and cut on buns. Pour water in the instant pot and insert the steamer rack.

3. Put the cinnamon rolls (buns) in the baking pan and transfer it on the rack. Close and seal the lid. Cook the dessert on manual mode (high pressure) for 20 minutes. Make a quick pressure release.

Nutritional info per serve: calories 173, fat 16.4, fiber 2.4, carbs 4.7, protein 3.1

Peanut Bars

Prep time: 25 minutes | **Cook time:** 12 minutes | **Yield:** 4 servings

Ingredients

- 2 tablespoons coconut oil
- 2 oz peanuts, chopped
- 2 tablespoons Swerve
- ½ teaspoon baking powder
- 4 tablespoons coconut flour
- 1 tablespoon butter, softened
- 1 teaspoon of cocoa powder
- 1 cup water, for cooking

Method

1. Make the pie crust: knead the dough from butter, coconut flour, and baking powder.

2. Then put the dough in the pie mold and flatten it. Pour water and insert the rack in the instant pot.

3. Put the pie crust in the instant pot. Close and seal the lid. Cook it on manual mode (high pressure) for 12 minutes. Make a quick pressure release.

4. Meanwhile, mix up peanuts, coconut oil, Swerve, and cocoa powder. Melt the mixture. When the pie crust is cooked, pour the peanut mixture over it and cool it.

Nutritional info per serve: calories 199, fat 17.5, fiber 4.3, carbs 8.8, protein 4.8

Frozen Strawberry Cheesecake

Prep time: 20 minutes | **Cook time:** 10 minutes | **Yield:** 2 servings

Ingredients

- 1 tablespoon gelatin
- 4 tablespoon water (for gelatin)
- 4 tablespoon cream cheese
- 1 strawberry, chopped
- ¼ cup of coconut milk
- 1 tablespoon swerve

Method

1. Mix up gelatin and water and leave the mixture for 10 minutes.

2. Meanwhile, pour coconut milk in the instant pot. Bring it to boil on saute mode (appx. For 10 minutes).

3. Meanwhile, mash the strawberry and mix it up with cream cheese.

4. Add the mixture in the hot coconut milk and stir until smooth.

5. Cool the liquid for 10 minutes and add gelatin. Whisk it until gelatin is melted.

6. Then pour the cheesecake in the mold and freeze in the freezer for 3 hours.

Nutritional info per serve: calories 155, fat 14.1, fiber 0.8, carbs 3.7, protein 5.2

Avocado Muffins

Prep time: 15 minutes | **Cook time:** 10 minutes | **Yield:** 3 servings

Ingredients

- 2 tablespoons almond flour
- 1 teaspoon flax meal
- 2 teaspoon swerve
- ¼ teaspoon baking powder
- 3 tablespoons coconut milk
- 2 eggs, beaten
- ½ avocado, mashed
- 1 cup of water (for instant pot)

Method

1. Whisk together the beaten egg, coconut milk, and baking powder.

2. Add swerve and flax meal.

3. After this, add almond flour, mashed avocado, and stir until homogenous.

4. Pour the batter into the muffin molds. Pour 1 cup of water in the instant pot and insert the steamer ramekin.

5. Transfer the muffins on the rack.

6. Set the "Manual" mode and put the timer on 10 minutes (High Pressure – QR for 10 minutes).

7. Cool the muffins to the room temperature.

Nutritional info per serve: calories 259, fat 22.6, fiber 4.8, carbs 9.7, protein 8.8

Nutmeg and Cinnamon Cake

Prep time: 15 minutes | **Cook time:** 10 minutes | **Yield:** 4 servings

Ingredients
- 1 teaspoon ground nutmeg
- ½ teaspoon ground cinnamon
- 1 egg, whisked
- 1/3 teaspoon baking powder
- ½ cup coconut flour
- 1 tablespoon almond butter
- ¼ cup of water
- 1 cup water (for instant pot)

Method
1. Stir together the whisked egg and water.
2. Add almond butter, coconut flour, baking powder, ground cinnamon, and ground nutmeg. Stir the mixture together until smooth and homogenous.
3. Transfer the dough into the non-stick cake pan and flatten it well with the help of the fingertips.
4. Pour 1 cup of water in the instant pot bowl and insert the trivet. Put the cake pan on the trivet and cover it with the foil.
5. Coo the cake on "Manual" mode (High pressure) for 10 minutes + NPR.

Nutritional info per serve: calories 104, fat 5, fiber 6.7, carbs 11.5, protein 4.3

Vanilla Liquid Cake

Prep time: 15 minutes | **Cook time:** 5 minutes | **Yield:** 2 servings

Ingredients
- ¼ teaspoon vanilla extract
- 2 eggs, whisked
- 3 tablespoon coconut oil
- ½ teaspoon baking powder
- 4 tablespoon coconut flour
- 2 tablespoons heavy cream

Method
1. Mix up vanilla extract and coconut oil.
2. After this, add whisked eggs, heavy cream, baking powder, and coconut flour.
3. Stir the mixture with the help of the fork until smooth texture.
4. Pour the batter into 2 small cake molds. Pour water in the instant pot and insert the cake molds.
5. Set "Manual" mode for 5 minutes (High pressure).
6. Allow the natural pressure release for 5 minutes more.

Nutritional info per serve: calories 363, fat 32.8, fiber 6, carbs 10.4, protein 8.9

Lime Mugs

Prep time: 15 minutes | **Cook time:** 15 minutes | **Yield:** 2 servings

Ingredients
- ½ cup of coconut milk
- ½ teaspoon lime zest, grated
- 1/3 teaspoon baking powder
- 4 tablespoons
- almond flour
- 1 egg yolk
- 1 tablespoon liquid stevia
- 1 cup water (for instant pot)

Method
1. Whisk the coconut milk gently and add lime zest. Add baking powder and almond flour.
2. After this, whisk the egg and add it to the coconut mixture. Add liquid stevia. Whisk the mixture until smooth and pour it into the mugs.
3. Cover the top of the mugs with the foil and make the small holes with the help of the toothpick.
4. Pour water into the instant pot and insert the steamer rack. Seal the lid and set the "steam" mode. Cook the cakes on "steam" mode for 13 minutes + quick pressure release. Chill the cakes for 5 minutes and discard the foil.

Nutritional info per serve: calories 250, fat 23.2, fiber 2.9, carbs 7.1, protein 5.7

Spiced Pudding

Prep time: 10 minutes | **Cook time:** 30 minutes | **Yield:** 2 servings

Ingredients
- 1 egg, beaten
- ¼ cup heavy cream
- 1 tablespoon Erythritol
- ¼ teaspoon pumpkin
- pie spices
- 1 teaspoon coconut oil
- 1 cup of water (for instant pot)

Method
1. Whisk the egg and mix it up with the heavy cream. Add Erythritol and pumpkin pie spices. Stir the mixture.
2. Grease the cake pan with the coconut oil and transfer the pudding mixture inside. Pour 1 cup of water in the instant pot.
3. Put the pudding on the steamer rack in the instant pot. Cover the pudding with the foil and secure edges. Put the "Manual" mode (High pressure) for 20 minutes.
4. Make the natural pressure release for 10 minutes. Chill the pudding for 10 hours before serving.

Nutritional info per serve: calories 101, fat 10, fiber 0, carbs 8.2, protein 3.1

Coconut Balls

Prep time: 5 minutes | **Cook time:** 8 minutes | **Yield:** 2 servings

Ingredients

- 2 tablespoon coconut flakes
- 1 egg, whisked
- 2 tablespoons coconut flour
- ¾ teaspoon vanilla extract
- 1 teaspoon Erythritol
- 1 tablespoon coconut oil
- 1 cup of water

Method

1. Combine together the whisked egg, coconut flour, coconut flakes, and vanilla extract. Add coconut oil. Add baking powder and Erythritol. Make the balls from the coconut flour mixture.

2. Pour 1 cup of water in the instant pot. Insert the steamer rack inside and place the ramekin on it. Add coconut balls.

3. Close and lock the instant pot lid. Set the "Manual" mode for 8 minutes – high pressure. (QPR). Chill the dessert for 5-10 minutes or until they are warm.

Nutritional info per serve: calories 142, fat 11.4, fiber 3.5, carbs 6.8, protein 3.9

Turnip Cake Cups

Prep time: 15 minutes | **Cook time:** 10 minutes | **Yield:** 2 servings

Ingredients

- 1 egg
- 1 tablespoon butter
- 1 teaspoon liquid stevia
- ¾ teaspoon vanilla extract
- ½ cup turnip, chopped
- 1 tablespoon macadamia nuts, crushed
- ¾ 2 tablespoons coconut flour
- ¾ teaspoon ground cinnamon
- ¾ teaspoon baking powder
- 1 cup of water

Method

1. Crack the egg in the mixing bowl and whisk it well with the help of the hand whisker. Add liquid stevia, vanilla extract, coconut flour, ground cinnamon, and baking powder. Stir well until smooth.

2. Then add macadamia nuts and turnip. Mix up the batter with the help of the spoon until homogenous. Pour the batter into the non-stick cake molds. Then pour 1 cup of water in the instant pot. Insert the steamer rack.

3. Transfer the cakes on the rack and close the instant pot lid. Seal the lid and set the "Manual" mode (High pressure) for 10 minutes. (QPR). Chill the cakes for 10-15 minutes

Nutritional info per serve: calories 147, fat 11.3, fiber 4.5, carbs 9.3, protein 4.5

Cardamom Rolls

Prep time: 20 minutes | **Cook time:** 18 minutes | **Yield:** 5 servings

Ingredients

- ½ cup coconut flour
- 1 tablespoon ground cardamom
- 2 tablespoon Splenda
- 1 egg, whisked
- ¼ cup almond milk
- 1 tablespoon butter, softened
- 1 tablespoon cream cheese
- 1/3 cup of water

Method

1. Combine coconut flour, almond milk, and softened butter. Knead the smooth dough. Roll up the dough with the help of the rolling pin.

2. Then combine together Erythritol and ground cardamom. Sprinkle the surface of the dough with the ground cardamom mixture.

3. Roll the dough into one big roll and cut them into servings. Place the rolls into the instant pot round mold. Pour water in the instant pot (1/3 cup) and insert the mold inside. Set "Manual" mode (High pressure) for 18 minutes.

4. Then use the natural pressure release method for 15 minutes. Chill the rolls to the room temperature and spread with cream cheese.

Nutritional info per serve: calories 128, fat 5.9, fiber 4.5, carbs 12.5, protein 5

Zebra Cakes in Cup

Prep time: 8 minutes | **Cook time:** 10 minutes | **Yield:** 3 servings

Ingredients

- 1 egg, whisked
- 2 tablespoons butter, melted
- 1 teaspoon Splenda
- 4 tablespoons almond flour
- 1 tablespoon cocoa powder
- 1 cup of water

Method

1. Mix up egg, butter, Splenda, and almond flour. Whisk the mixture until smooth. Then separate the liquid into halves. Pour white liquid into the baking cups.

2. Add the cocoa in the remaining white batter and whisk until it turns the color into chocolate. Add the chocolate liquid in the baking cups too and gently stir to get the zebra stripes.

3. Pour 1 cup of water in the instant pot. Place the steamer rack. Transfer the cups on the steamer rack and close the lid. Seal the instant pot lid and set the "Manual" mode. Put the timer for 9 minutes (Quick pressure release). When the dessert is cooked – let it chill for 1 hour.

Nutritional info per serve: calories 313, fat 28.1, fiber 4.5, carbs 10.4, protein 10.3

Measurement Conversion Charts

Measurement

Cup	Ounces	Milliliters	Tablespoons
8 cups	64 oz	1895	128
6 cups	48 oz	1420	96
5 cups	40 oz	1180	80
4 cups	32 oz	960	64
2 cups	16 oz	480	32
1 cups	8 oz	240	16
3/4 cups	6 oz	177	12
2/3 cups	5 oz	158	11
1/2 cups	4 oz	118	8
3/8 cups	3 oz	90	6
1/3 cups	2.5 oz	79	5.5
1/4 cups	2 oz	59	4
1/8 cups	1 oz	30	3
1/16 cups	1/2 oz	15	1

Weight

Imperial	Metric
1/2 oz	15 g
1 oz	29 g
2 oz	57 g
3 oz	85 g
4 oz	113 g
5 oz	141 g
6 oz	170 g
8 oz	227 g
10 oz	283 g
12 oz	340 g
13 oz	369 g
14 oz	397 g
15 oz	425 g
1 lb	453 g

Temperature

Fahrenheit	Celsius
100 °F	37 °C
150 °F	65 °C
200 °F	93 °C
250 °F	121 °C
300 °F	150 °C
325 °F	160 °C
350 °F	180 °C
375 °F	190 °C
400 °F	200 °C
425 °F	220 °C
450 °F	230 °C
500 °F	260 °C
525 °F	274 °C
550 °F	288 °C

Recipe Index

Portobello Cheese Sandwiches, 144

cheese (Feta)
Feta Chicken Drumsticks, 117
Red Feta Soup, 62
Salmon Salad with Feta, 51
Feta Psiti, 43
Feta Stuffed Chicken, 26

cheese (Mascarpone)
Butter Chicken, 106
Mascarpone Tilapia, 134
Bang Bang Shrimps, 124
Chicken Pasta, 107
Crack Chicken, 104
Peppercorn Pork, 92

cheese (Monterey Jack)
3-Cheese Quiche Cups, 33
Big Mac Salad, 78
Jalapenos with Cheese, 36
Cheeseburger Soup, 57
Chicken Pasta, 107
Jalapeno Soup, 64
Leek Soup, 151
Pork Florentine, 85
Rangoon Crab Dip, 46
Stuffed Mushrooms, 39
Steamed Spinach with Garlic, 43

cheese (Mozzrella)
3-Cheese Quiche Cups, 33
Beef Bake with Chives, 80
Buffalo Style Soup, 67
Cheese Bombs, 45
Egg Cups, 21
Eggplant Lasagna, 98
Eggplant Parm, 47
Low Carb Pot Pie, 114
Margherita Egg Cups, 25
Mozzarella Fish Sticks, 130
Mozzarella Stuffed Meatballs, 94
Omelet "3-Cheese", 32
Pizza Soup, 61
Pork Quiche, 101
Salmon Caprese, 126

Sausage Balls, 38
Spinach Dip, 37
Taco Bites, 38
Tender Turkey Tetrazzini, 110
Chicken Lombardy, 112
Cordon Blue Soup, 67
Crustless Fish Pie, 129

cheese (Parmesan)
Bacon Casserole, 26
Bacon Deviled Eggs, 36
Cauliflower Fritters, 42
Cheese Roll-Ups, 24
Chicken Carbonara, 116
Chicken Lombardy, 112
Garlic Asparagus, 48
Haddock Bake, 135
Mushroom Mini Pizza, 112
Paprika Zucchini Soup, 66
Parm Zucchini Noodles, 139
Parmesan Balls with Greens, 41
Parmesan Chicken Fillets, 106
Pork Milanese, 92
Salmon Loaf, 130
Stuffed Pork Rolls, 87
Tender Turkey Tetrazzini, 110
Zucchini Fries, 45
Brussel Sprouts Hash, 48

cheese (Pecorino)
Pecorino Chicken Cubes, 121
Vegetable Frittata, 28

cheese (Provolone)
Cauliflower Soup, 57
Cheese Jalapenos, 30
Morning Aromatic Casserole, 29
Omelet "3-Cheese", 32
Provolone Stuffed Chicken, 113
Reuben Pickles, 41
Sausage Puffs, 28
Stuffed Hard-Boiled Eggs, 23
Tuna Stuffed Poblanos, 134
Vegetable Lasagna with Meat, 83

cheese (Ricotta)
Cordon Blue Soup, 67
Portobello Steak, 145
Zucchini Ravioli, 47

cheese (Romano)
Romano Pork Chops, 92

cheese (Swiss)
Quail Egg Bites, 31
chicken
Breakfast Casserole, 20
Breakfast Sandwich, 22
Buffalo Style Soup, 67
Cheese Chicken Kofte, 111
Chicken Carbonara, 116
Chicken Fritters, 116
Chicken Slaw Mix, 114
Chicken Zucchini Rings, 116
Greek Burger, 110
Herbed Whole Chicken, 107
Meat and Cauliflower Bake, 24
Mushroom Mini Pizza, 112
Parmesan Balls with Greens, 41
"Ramen" Soup, 62
Aromatic Eggplant Mix, 53
Bacon Chicken, 120
Bacon-Wrapped Tenders, 115
Beef Stuffed Kale, 80
Bok Choy Soup, 65
Broccoli Cheese Soup, 56
Butter Chicken, 106
Cabbage Soup, 57
Celery Salad with Chicken, 118
Celery Stalk Chicken Salad, 5
Cheesy Cream Soup, 59
Chicken Alfredo, 106
Chicken Celery Sticks, 116
Chicken Cubes in Succulent Sauce, 117
Chicken Curry with Cilantro, 108
Chicken Divan, 116
Chicken Drumsticks de Provance, 120